Managing Data in SPSS
– A Step by Step Guide
For Medical Researchers

Dr Sandheep Sugathan

MBBS MD DPH

Universiti Kuala Lumpur Royal College of Medicine Perak

1

Contents

PART I – Approaching your Data

Chapter 1

Steps in DATA ENTRY for Medical Researchers

Data entry is done after collection of data. Data entry is the first step for analysing your data.

Steps in data entry are as follows

1. Data cleansing and verification of data before entry
   - Making sure that all data, which are collected are correct and in a good format.
2. Coding of data
   - Multiple choices – categorical variables – nominal variables - Code as 1,2,3,…
     (For example ethnicity – Malay, Chinese, Indian and others)
   - Dichotomous responses – True or false / Correct or Incorrect / Present or Absent – Code as 1 and 0.
   - Good or Poor – Code as 1 and 0.
3. If some of your questions have multiple answers (example – what all diseases a person is suffering from?)
   It is better to key in each response as Yes or No (1 for yes and 0 for No)

Data can be entered either in

- Microsoft Excel or
- SPSS

If data is entered in MS Excel

- List out the variable names
  - Serial No.
  - Age
  - Gender
  - Ethnicity
  - Religion
  - Education
  - Occupation
  - Height
  - Weight
  - BMI

- Enter variable names in 1st row. Never merge first row with second row (that may create problems when you transfer data in MS Excel to SPSS)
- Enter each participant's or patient's information in each row.
- Make sure that the values key in are correct
- Make sure that spelling is correct
- After entering the data, save Excel Workbook in Excel 97 – 2003 Workbook format (.xls format). This is very important. If you save in Excel workbook format, sometimes SPSS may not be able to open the excel file.
- You must close the Excel Workbook after saving before you try to open in SPSS

- Open SPSS in your computer from
  Start menu ------ all programs

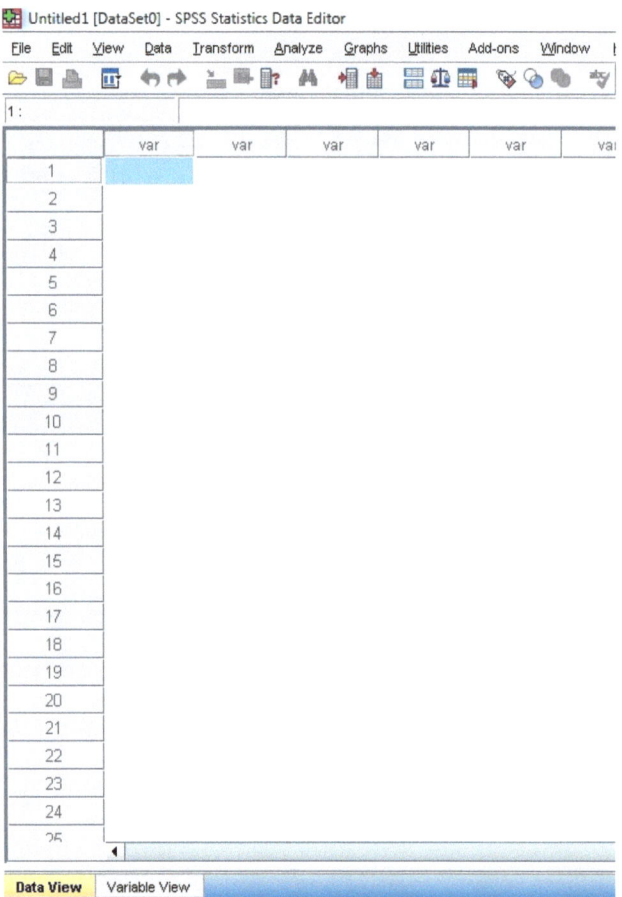

- Open File menu in SPSS Statistics Data Editor Window

- File ……………………. Open ………………………..Data

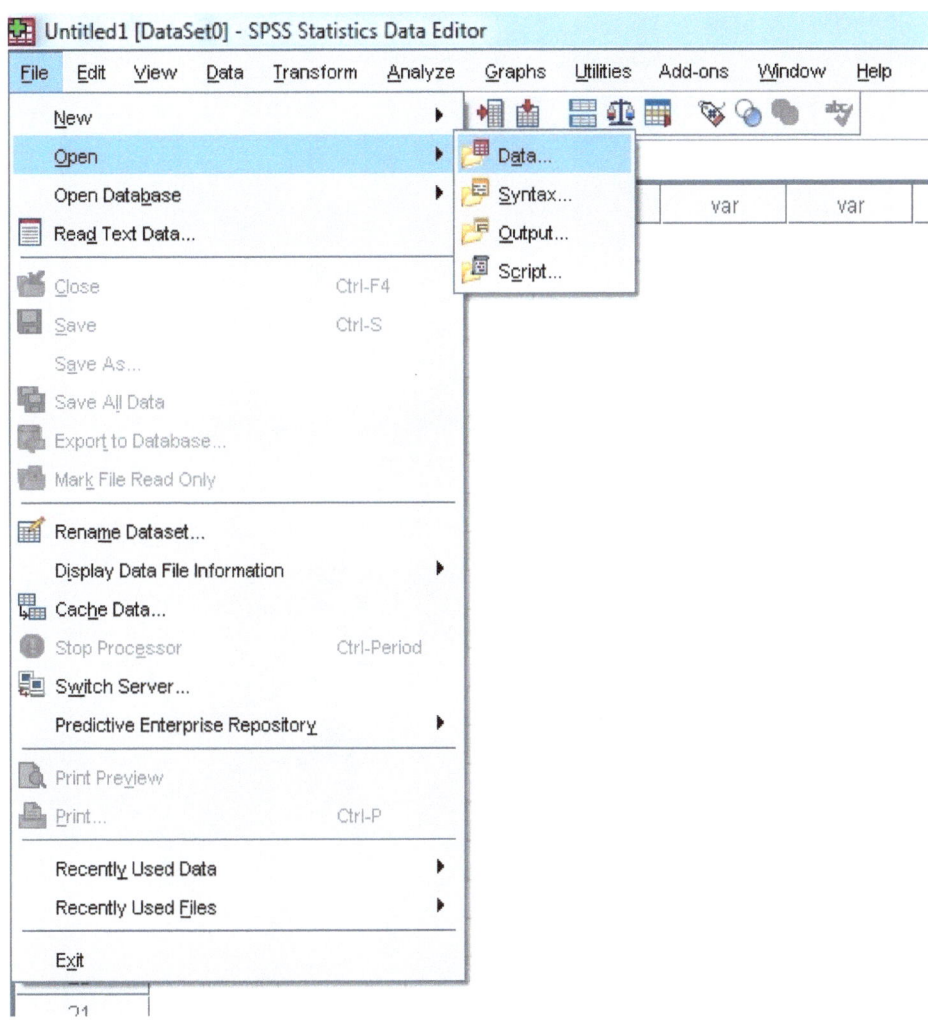

Select the destination, from where to open the data file (excel file to be opened)

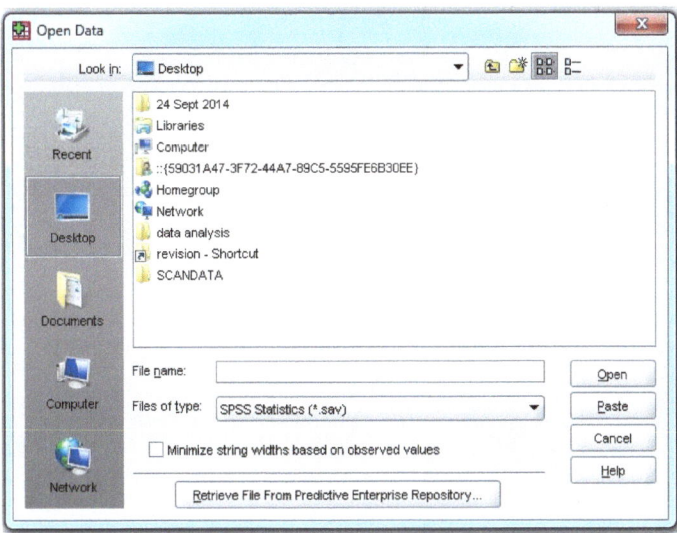

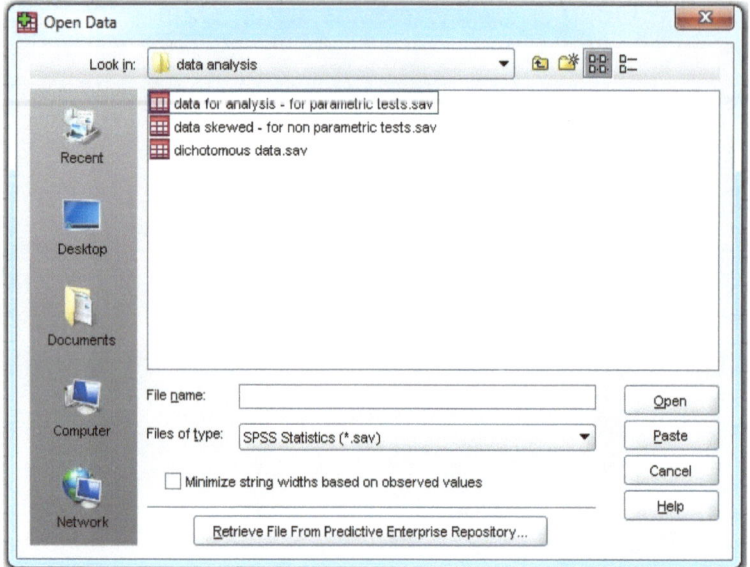

By default, the SPSS files in the folder will be shown.

Select the files of type to open as Excel (.xls).

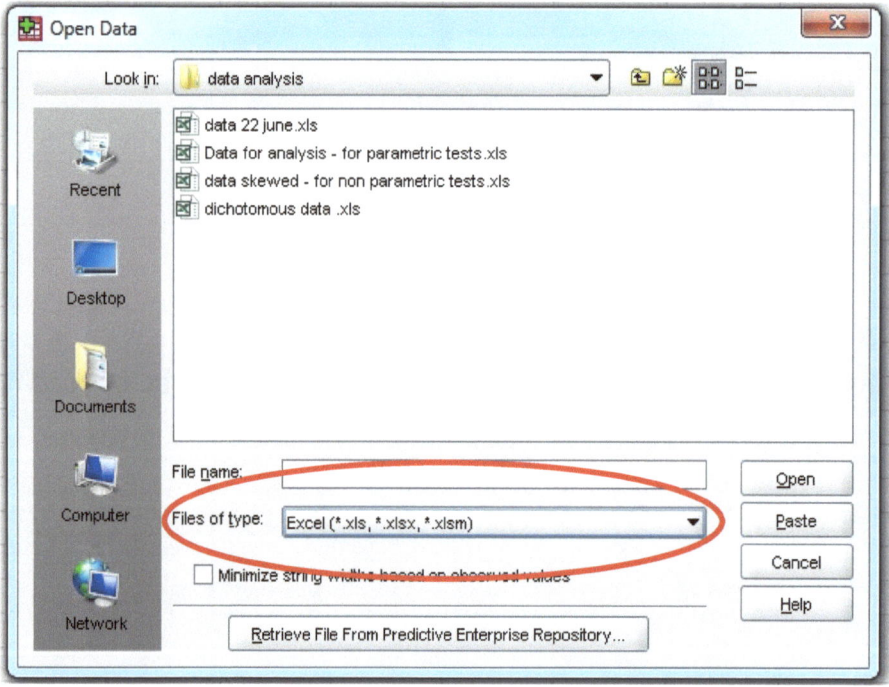

Then select the Excel file to be opened

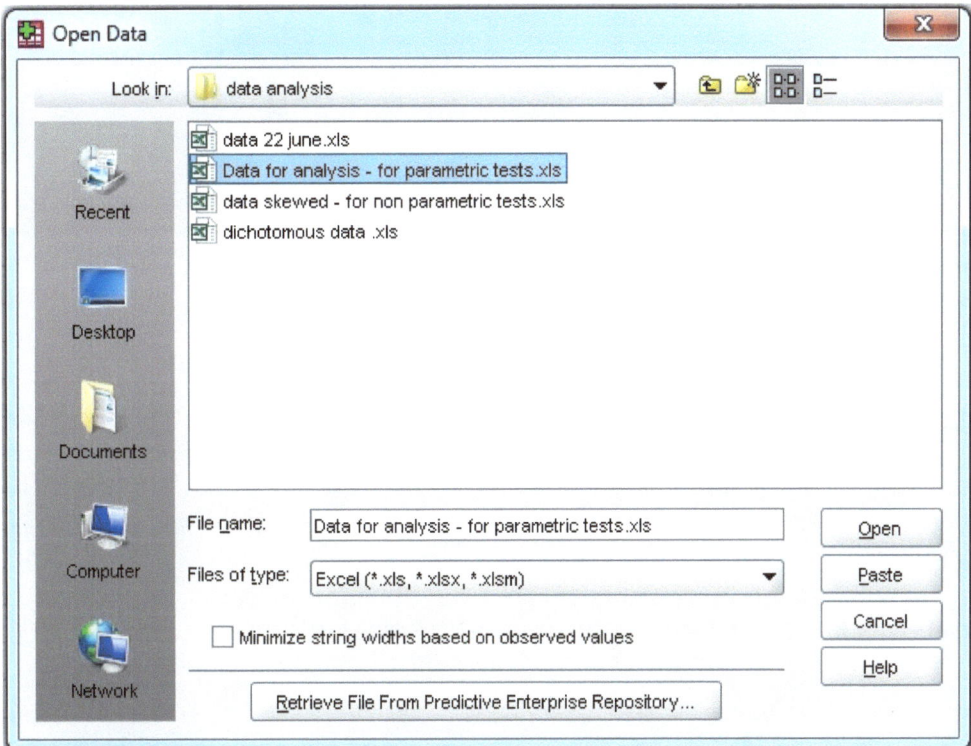

Then click Open.

Then a dialogue box appears as follows

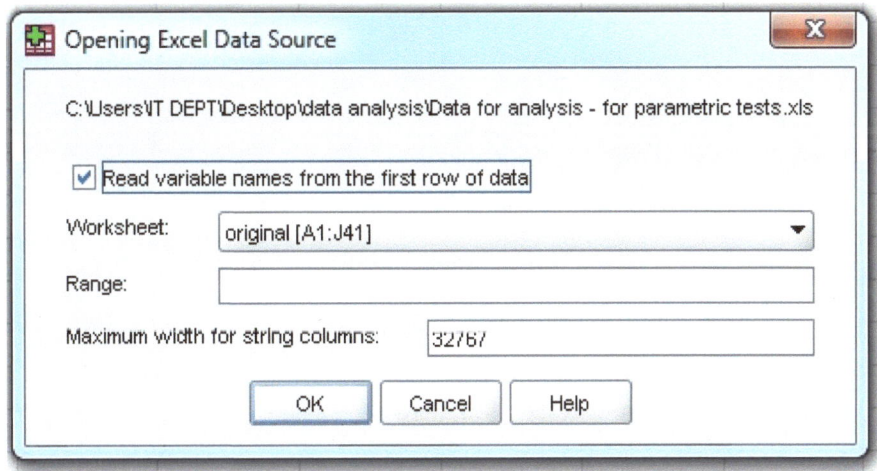

Select "Read variable names from the first row of data"

Select the worksheet of MS Excel which is to be opened

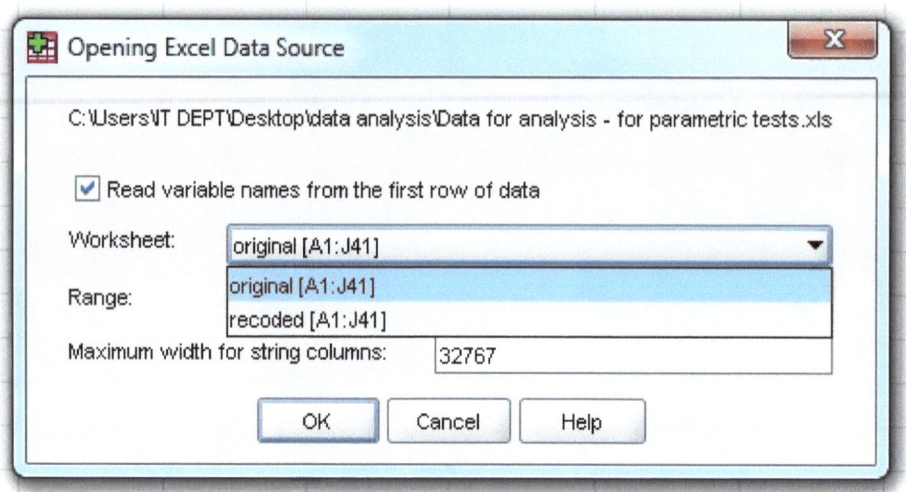

Then Click Ok

Then data from MS Excel will be imported to SPSS data editor

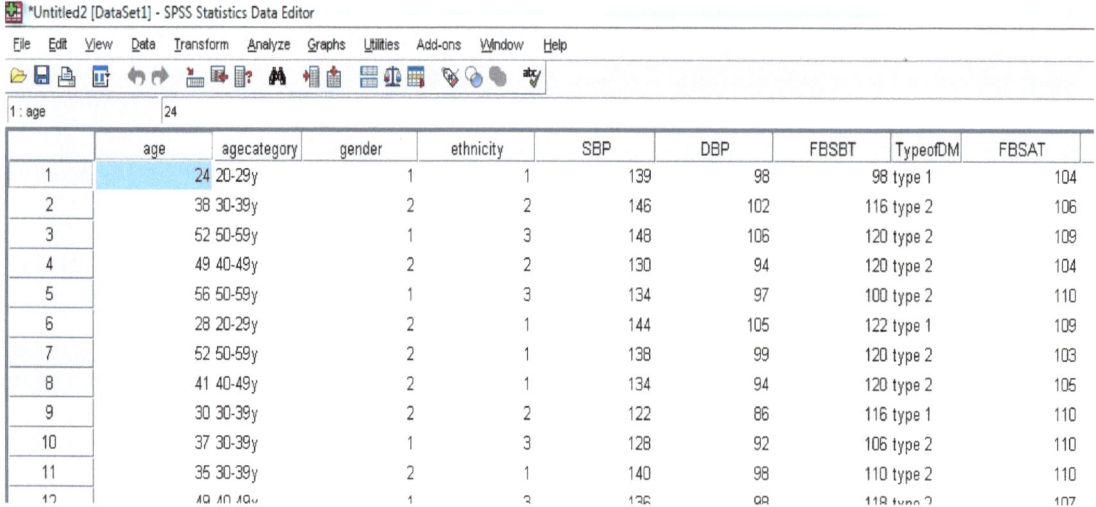

Click Variable view at the left bottom corner of the window

16	44 40-49y
17	22 20-29y
18	40 40-49y
19	43 40-49y
20	49 40-49y
21	59 50-59
22	36 30-39y
23	63 above 60
24	48 40-49y
25	36 30-39y

Data View   Variable View

Print

SPSS Data Editor Variable view opens

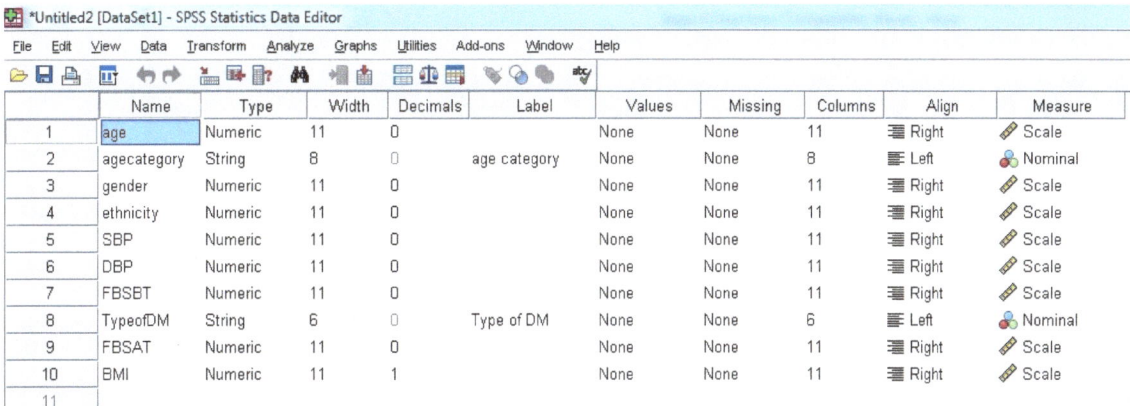

You can edit the characteristics of each variables in variable view.

1. Variable names – enter name without space in between

2. Variable types – Numeric when variable contains only numbers

   String type – when variables contain alphabet or numerals or alphanumerals

3. Width can be adjusted based on the number of digits or number of alphabets.

4. Decimels – Number of decimels you want, can be entered

5. Label – the variable. (You can give the preferred variable name)

6. Values for each number can be given

   Eg:- 1 for male and 2 for female

Name	Type	Width	Decimals	Label	Values	Missing	Columns	Align	Measure
age	Numeric	11	0		None	None	11	Right	Scale
agecategory	String	8	0	age category	None	None	8	Left	Nominal
gendor	Numeric	11	0		None	None	11	Right	Scale
ethnicity	Numeric	11	0		None	None	11	Right	Scale
SBP	Numeric	11	0		None	None	11	Right	Scale
DBP	Numeric	11	0		None	None	11	Right	Scale
FBSBT	Numeric	11	0						
TypeofDM	String	6	0	Type of [					
FBSAT	Numeric	11	0						
BMI	Numeric	11	1						

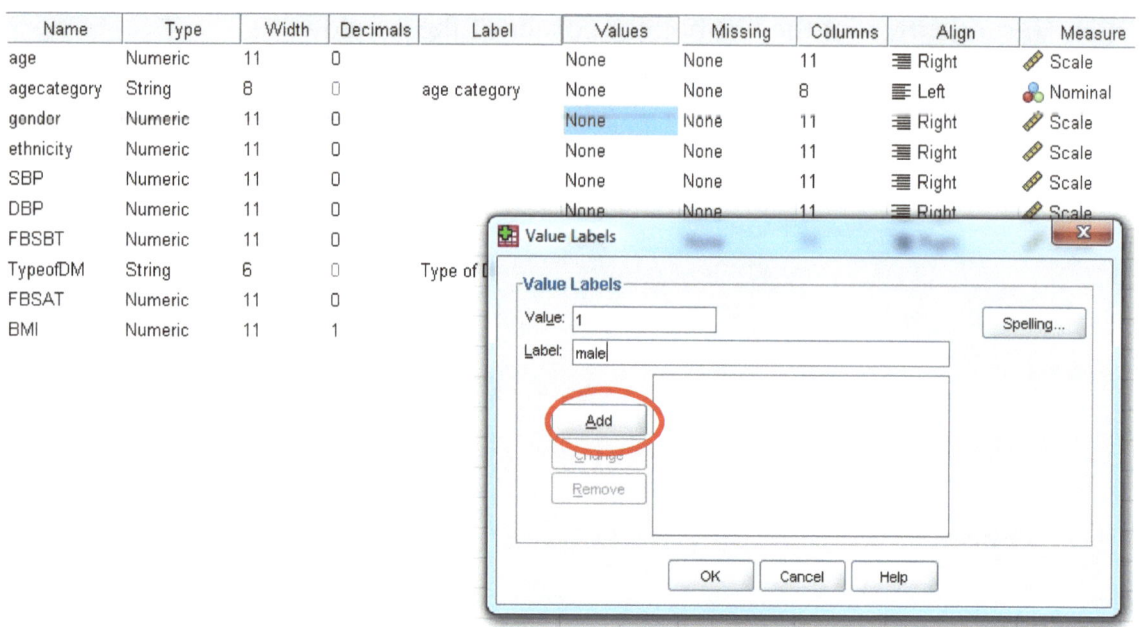

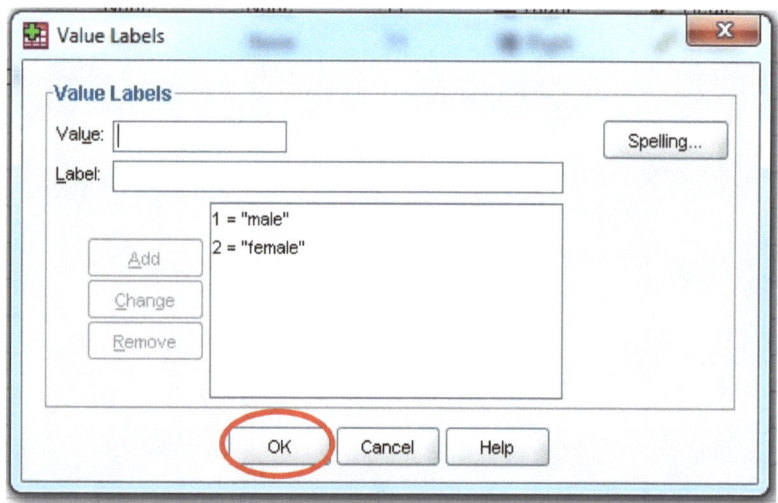

Enter the value. Click label for that value. Add. Then Click OK

7. Alignment (Left, Right or Centre)

8. Measure (Scale for continuous variables; Nominal or Ordinal)

Now your data is ready for analysis in SPSS

If you are entering the data directly in SPSS (not keying in MS Excel first)

1. Do coding before keying in the data

2. Define the variables in variable view

3. Enter the data

4. Do data cleansing to make sure that all the data are entered correctly.

How to convert continuous data to categorical data in SPSS?

Untitled2 [DataSet2] - SPSS Statistics D		

File   Edit   View   Data   Transform   A

4 :

	age	v
1	30	
2	31	
3	40	
4	42	
5	31	
6	36	
7	25	
8	32	
9	26	
10	28	
11	55	
12	35	
13	41	
14	25	
15	28	
16	22	
17	18	
18	27	
19	18	
20	18	
21	30	
22	29	

You are having a data of age of patients. Now you need to categorize age into 4 groups. (< 30 y, 30-39 y, 40-49y, ≥ 50 y).

Click Transform – recode into different variables

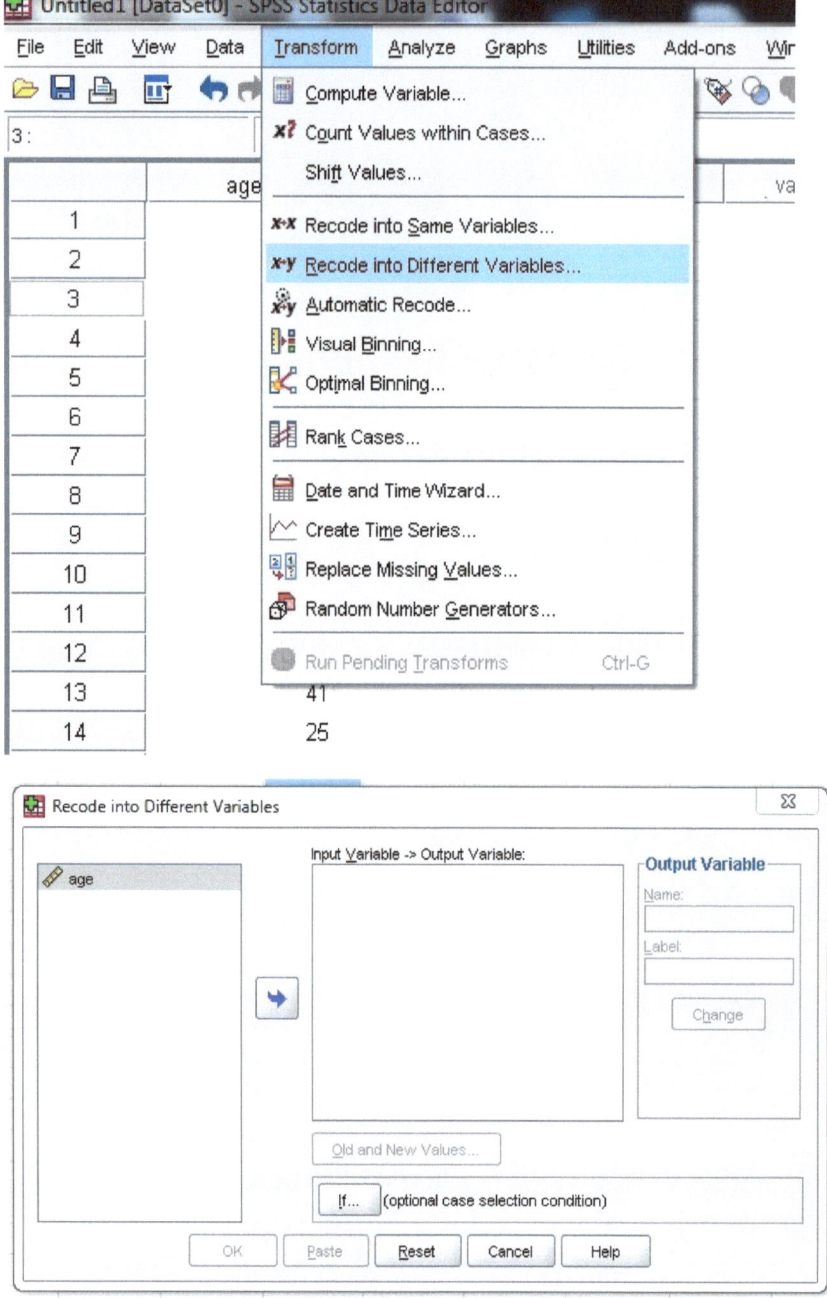

Put the continuous variable to be converted to categorical variable as the input variable.

Name the output variable (Name of the categorical variable). Click Change

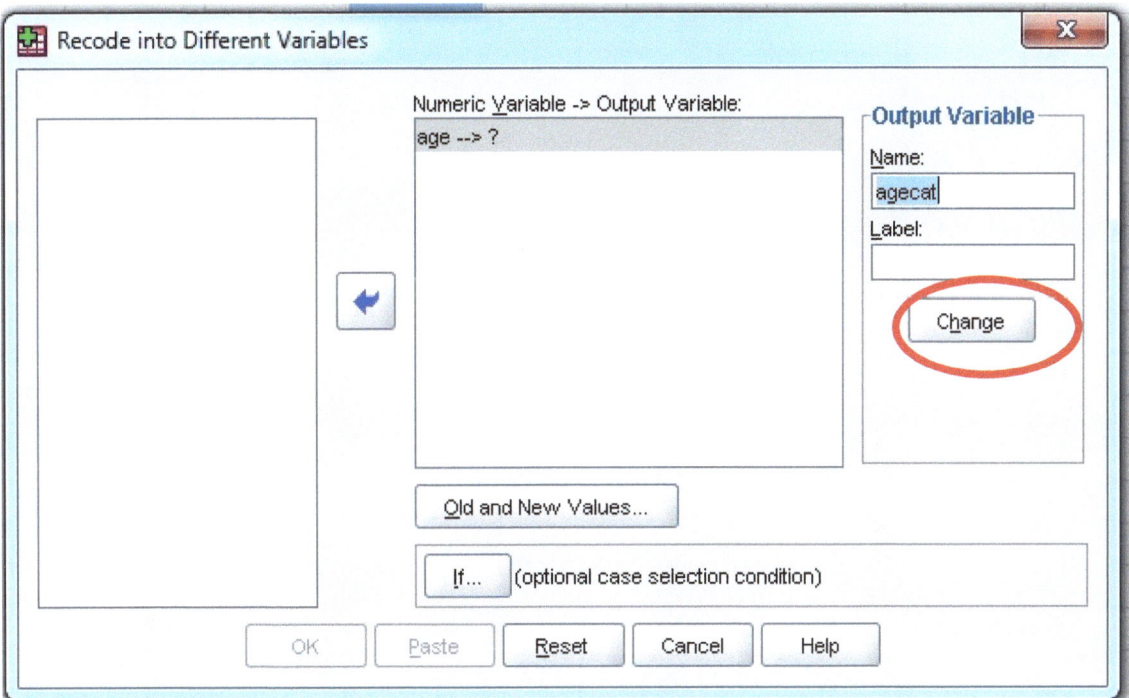

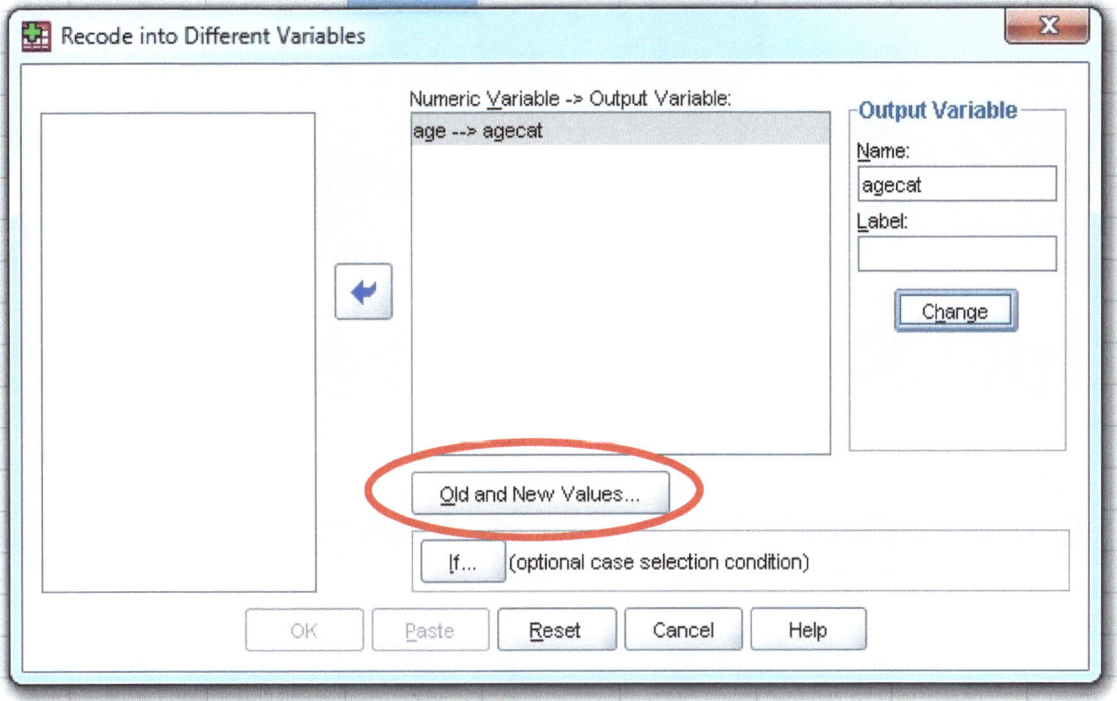

Click Old and New Values

Old values

 all age which are < 30 years – give new value 1 (Range, LOWEST through value – 29) – it will select all values 29 years and below

30 – 39 years ----------------- new value 2 (Range 30 through 39)

40 – 49 years ---------------- new value 3 (Range 40 through 49)

≥ 50 years -------------------- new value 4 (Range, value through HIGHEST – 50)

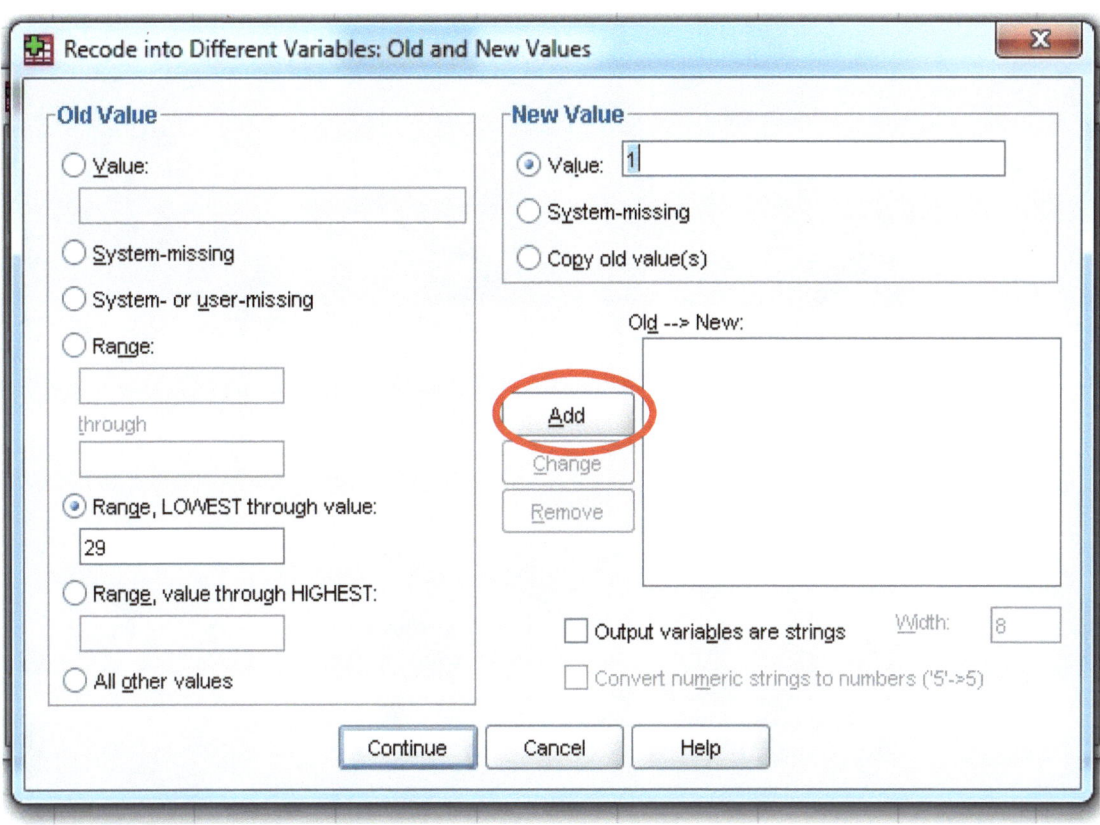

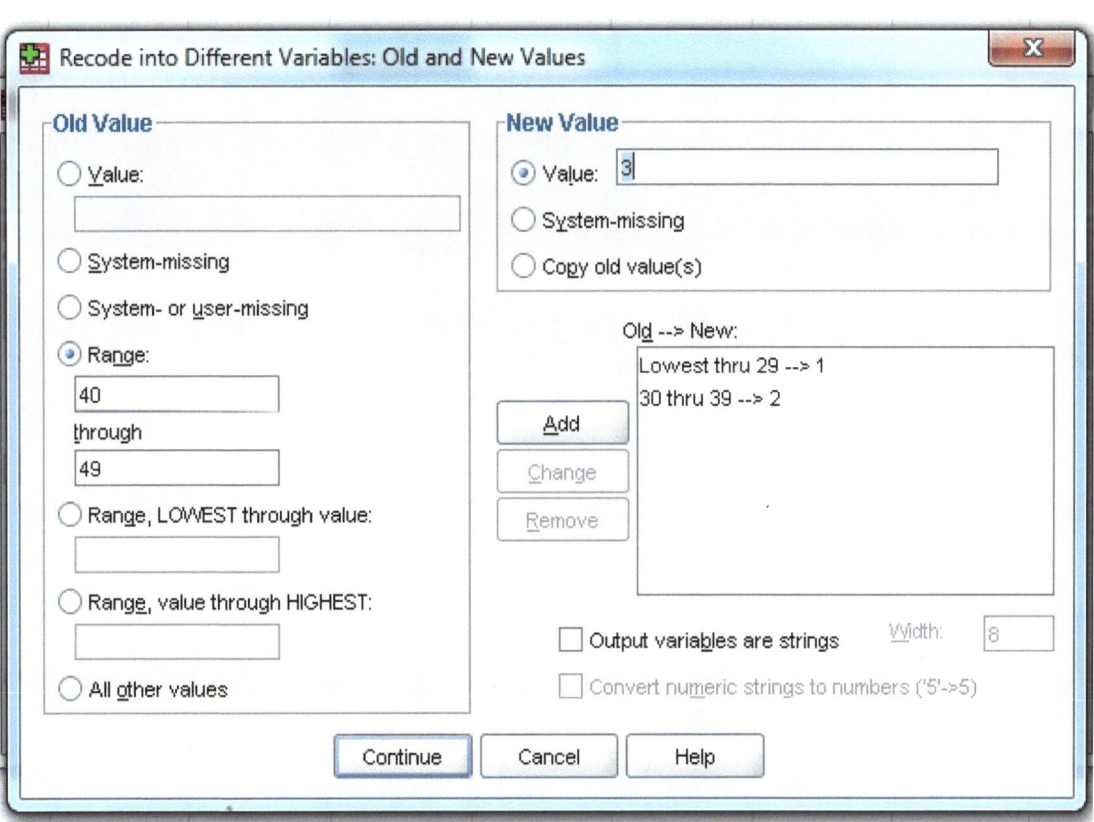

Recode into Different Variables: Old and New Values

Old Value
- ○ Value:
- ○ System-missing
- ○ System- or user-missing
- ○ Range:
  - through
- ○ Range, LOWEST through value:
- ◉ Range, value through HIGHEST:
  - 50
- ○ All other values

New Value
- ◉ Value: 4
- ○ System-missing
- ○ Copy old value(s)

Old --> New:
```
Lowest thru 29 --> 1
30 thru 39 --> 2
40 thru 49 --> 3
```
Add
Change
Remove

☐ Output variables are strings   Width: 8
☐ Convert numeric strings to numbers ('5'->5)

Continue   Cancel   Help

Recode into Different Variables: Old and New Values

Old Value
- ○ Value:
- ○ System-missing
- ○ System- or user-missing
- ○ Range:
  - through
- ○ Range, LOWEST through value:
- ◉ Range, value through HIGHEST:
- ○ All other values

New Value
- ◉ Value:
- ○ System-missing
- ○ Copy old value(s)

Old --> New:
```
Lowest thru 29 --> 1
30 thru 39 --> 2
40 thru 49 --> 3
50 thru Highest --> 4
```
Add
Change
Remove

☐ Output variables are strings   Width: 8
☐ Convert numeric strings to numbers ('5'->5)

Continue   Cancel   Help

After defining all the new values ----- Click continue

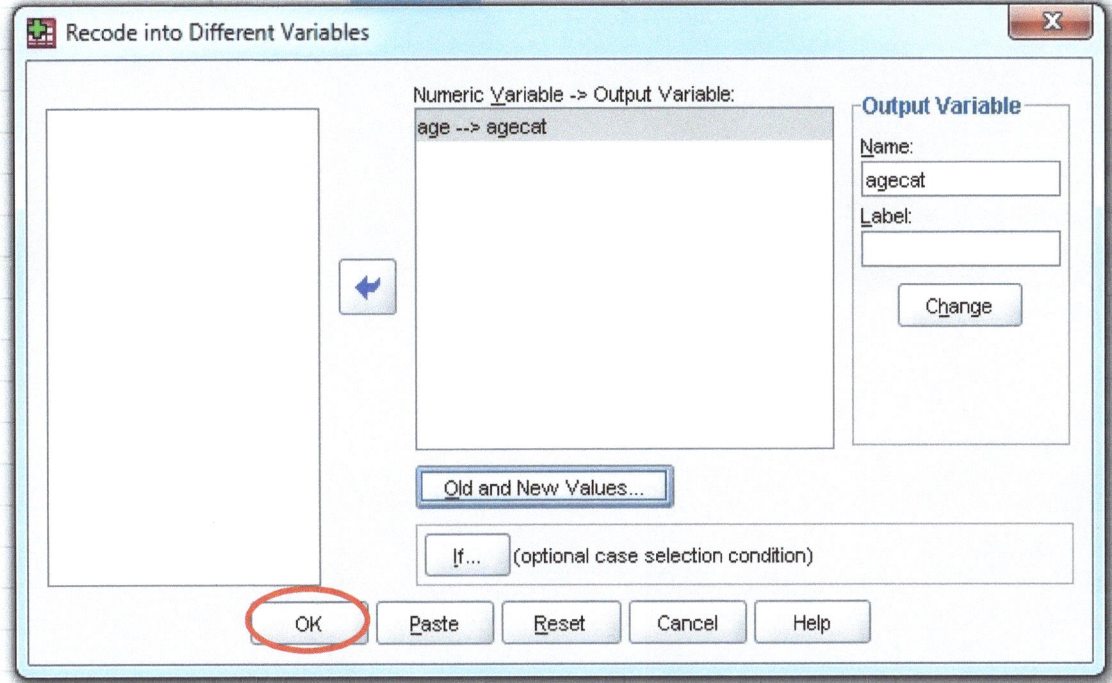

Click OK

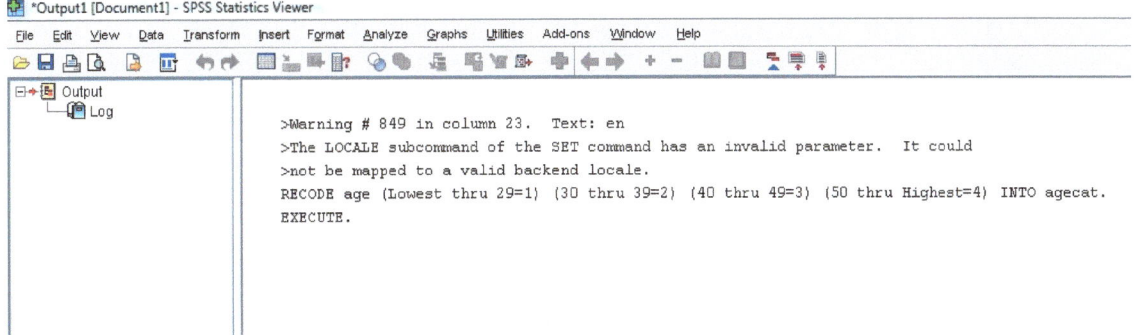

Output SPSS Statistics Viewer appears with message EXECUTE

Open SPSS Data Editor

One new category is created as the last column.

Untitled1 [DataSet0] - SPSS Statistics Data Editor

File Edit View Data Transform Analyze Graphs

	age	agecat
1	30	2.00
2	31	2.00
3	40	3.00
4	42	3.00
5	31	2.00
6	36	2.00
7	25	1.00
8	32	2.00
9	26	1.00
10	28	1.00
11	55	4.00
12	35	2.00
13	41	3.00
14	25	1.00
15	28	1.00
16	22	1.00
17	18	1.00
18	27	1.00

Coding of study to assess Knowledge

- Code each knowledge questions as 1 or 0 (1 will be for correct answer, 0 will be for wrong answer)
- Add all the knowledge questions scores – to get total knowledge score
- Categorize as poor knowledge or good knowledge based on total knowledge scores.
- 2 ways to categorize total knowledge score – less than median as poor, median and above as good
- Less than 25th percentile as poor, 25th percentile to 75th percentile including both as average, more than 75th percentile as good.

How to take total knowledge score using Excel

Open the MS Excel file, in which you key in the knowledge scores

				f_x				
A	B	C	D	E	F	G	H	
Sl No	K1	K2	K3	K4	K5	K6		
1	1	1	1	0	1	0		
2	1	0	0	1	0	0		
3	1	0	1	0	0	1		
4	0	1	0	1	1	0		
5	1	0	0	1	0	0		
6	1	0	1	1	1	1		
7	0	0	0	0	1	0		
8	1	1	0	0	0	1		
9	0	1	0	1	0	0		
10	1	0	1	1	1	0		
11	1	0	0	0	0	1		
12	1	1	1	1	1	0		
13	1	1	1	1	0	0		
14	0	0	0	1	0	1		
15	1	0	1	0	1	0		

Then you give a category as Total Knowledge Score (TKS) as a column at the end of last knowledge question (here K6).

Sl No	K1	K2	K3	K4	K5	K6	TKS
1	1	1	1	0	1	0	
2	1	0	0	1	0	0	
3	1	0	1	0	0	1	
4	0	1	0	1	1	0	
5	1	0	0	1	0	0	
6	1	0	1	1	1	1	
7	0	0	0	0	1	0	
8	1	1	0	0	0	1	
9	0	1	0	1	0	0	
10	1	0	1	1	1	0	
11	1	0	0	0	0	1	
12	1	1	1	1	1	0	
13	1	1	1	1	0	0	
14	0	0	0	1	0	1	
15	1	0	1	0	1	0	

Then you give formula for sum =sum(starting cell:ending cell)

A	B	C	D	E	F	G	H	I
Sl No	K1	K2	K3	K4	K5	K6	TKS	
1	1	1	1	0	1	0	=sum(B2:G2)	
2	1	0	0	1	0	0		
3	1	0	1	0	0	1		
4	0	1	0	1	1	0		
5	1	0	0	1	0	0		
6	1	0	1	1	1	1		
7	0	0	0	0	1	0		
8	1	1	0	0	0	1		
9	0	1	0	1	0	0		
10	1	0	1	1	1	0		
11	1	0	0	0	0	1		
12	1	1	1	1	1	0		
13	1	1	1	1	0	0		
14	0	0	0	1	0	1		
15	1	0	1	0	1	0		

After giving the formula for sum, close the bracket and click enter

Then sum of all the selected cells appear.

SI No	K1	K2	K3	K4	K5	K6	TKS
1	1	1	1	0	1	0	4
2	1	0	0	1	0	0	
3	1	0	1	0	0	1	
4	0	1	0	1	1	0	
5	1	0	0	1	0	0	
6	1	0	1	1	1	1	
7	0	0	0	0	1	0	
8	1	1	0	0	0	1	
9	0	1	0	1	0	0	
10	1	0	1	1	1	0	
11	1	0	0	0	0	1	
12	1	1	1	1	1	0	
13	1	1	1	1	0	0	
14	0	0	0	1	0	1	
15	1	0	1	0	1	0	

Now you select the cell showing sum of first row. Then drag it down from the right down corner of the cell. So sum of all the rows will appear, to give you TKS (total knowledge score) of all the rows.

SI No	K1	K2	K3	K4	K5	K6	TKS
1	1	1	1	0	1	0	4
2	1	0	0	1	0	0	2
3	1	0	1	0	0	1	3
4	0	1	0	1	1	0	3
5	1	0	0	1	0	0	2
6	1	0	1	1	1	1	5
7	0	0	0	0	1	0	1
8	1	1	0	0	0	1	3
9	0	1	0	1	0	0	2
10	1	0	1	1	1	0	4
11	1	0	0	0	0	1	2
12	1	1	1	1	1	0	5
13	1	1	1	1	0	0	4
14	0	0	0	1	0	1	2
15	1	0	1	0	1	0	3

You can take the total knowledge score using SPSS also

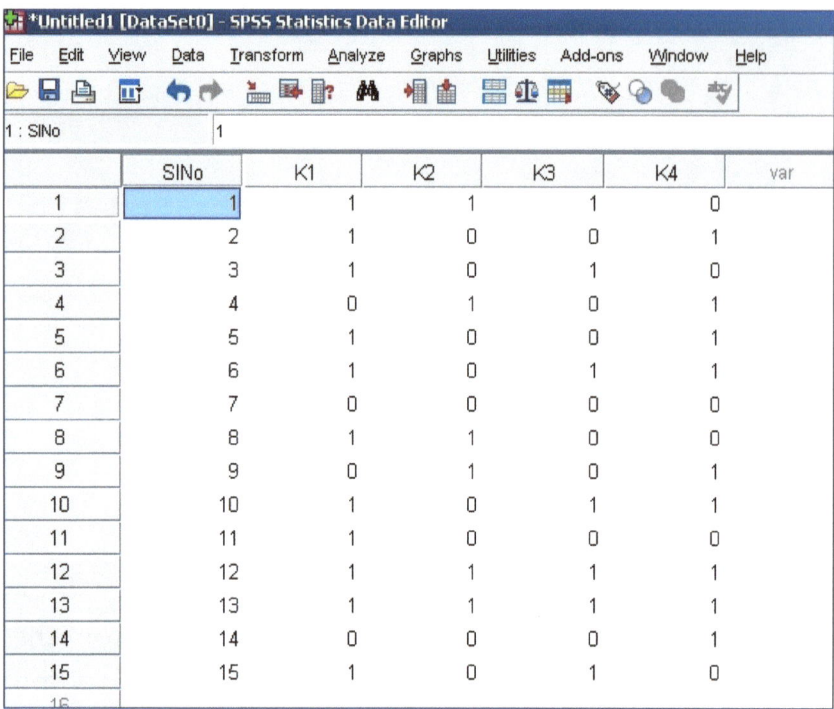

Select Transform ---------- Compute Variable

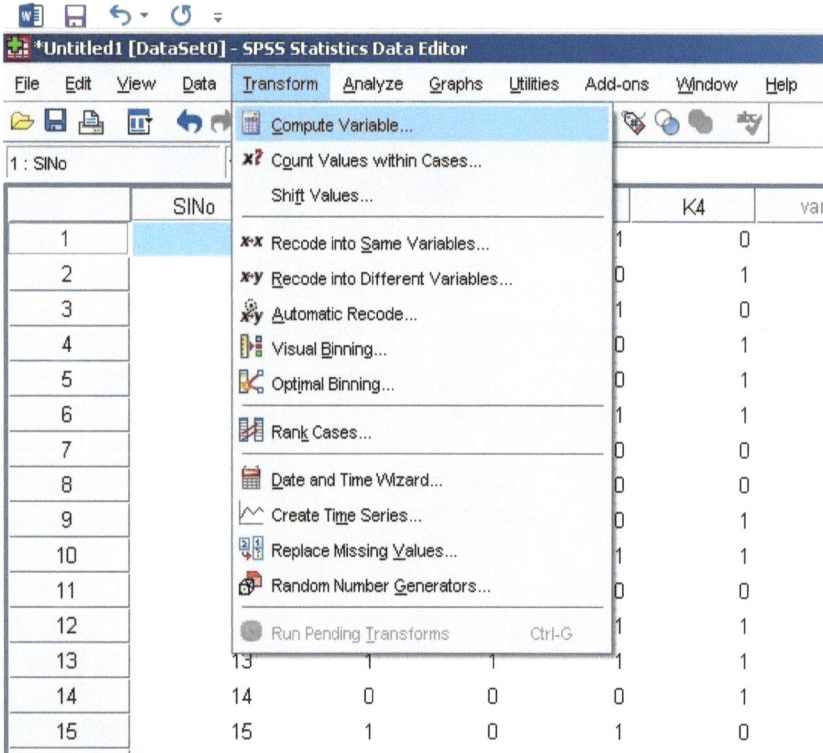

Then a message box appears like below.

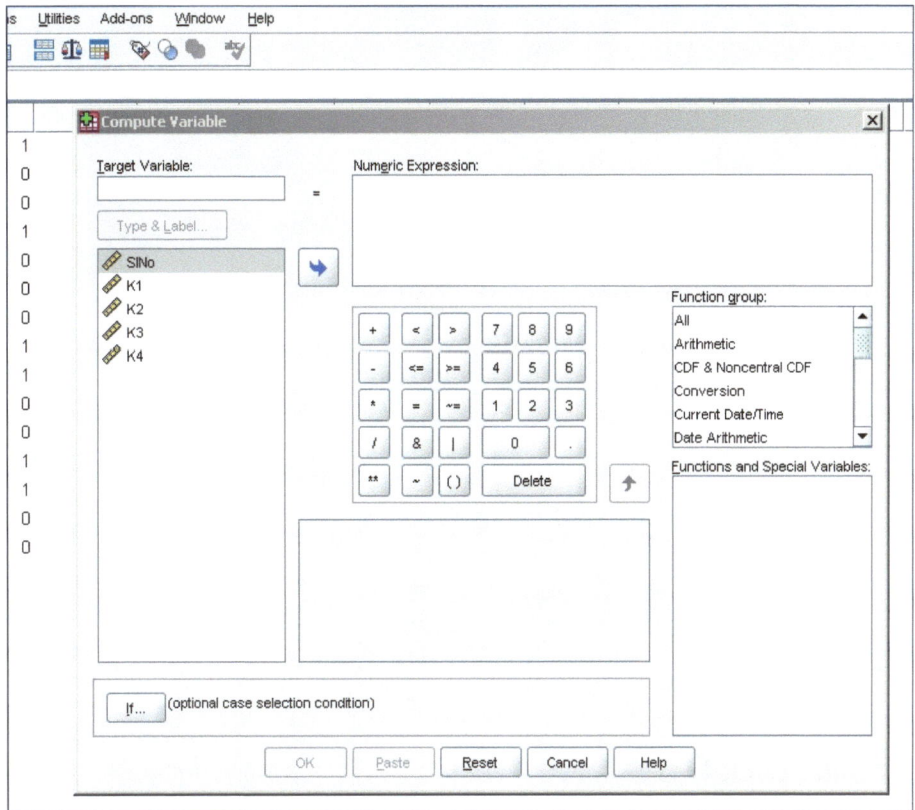

Name the target variable (for example here we will type as TKS that is total knowledge score)

Numeric expression can be given. That is the formula to get total knowledge score.

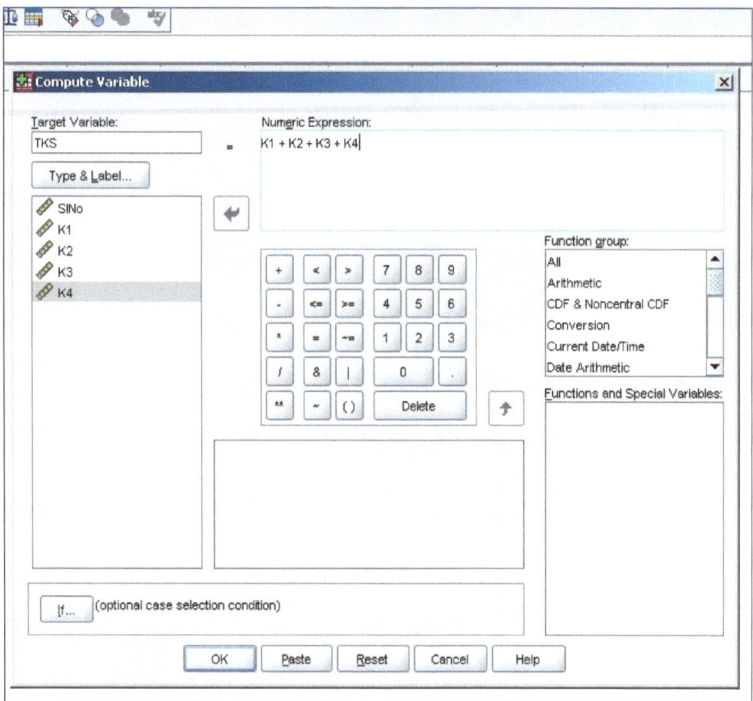

After giving the formula, click OK

Then in SPSS Data Editor, a new column will be added at the last as TKS

SINo	K1	K2	K3	K4	TKS
1	1	1	1	0	3.00
2	1	0	0	1	2.00
3	1	0	1	0	2.00
4	0	1	0	1	2.00
5	1	0	0	1	2.00
6	1	0	1	1	3.00
7	0	0	0	0	.00
8	1	1	0	0	2.00
9	0	1	0	1	2.00
10	1	0	1	1	3.00
11	1	0	0	0	1.00
12	1	1	1	1	4.00
13	1	1	1	1	4.00
14	0	0	0	1	1.00
15	1	0	1	0	2.00

Data entry should be done always, keeping in mind your objectives and data analysis.

PART II – Analyzing your Data

Chapter 2

DESCRIPTIVE STATISTICS OF CONTINUOUS VARIABLES USING SPSS

Method 1 for descriptive statistics of continuous variables

Click Analyze ---------- Descriptive Statistics -------------- Frequencies

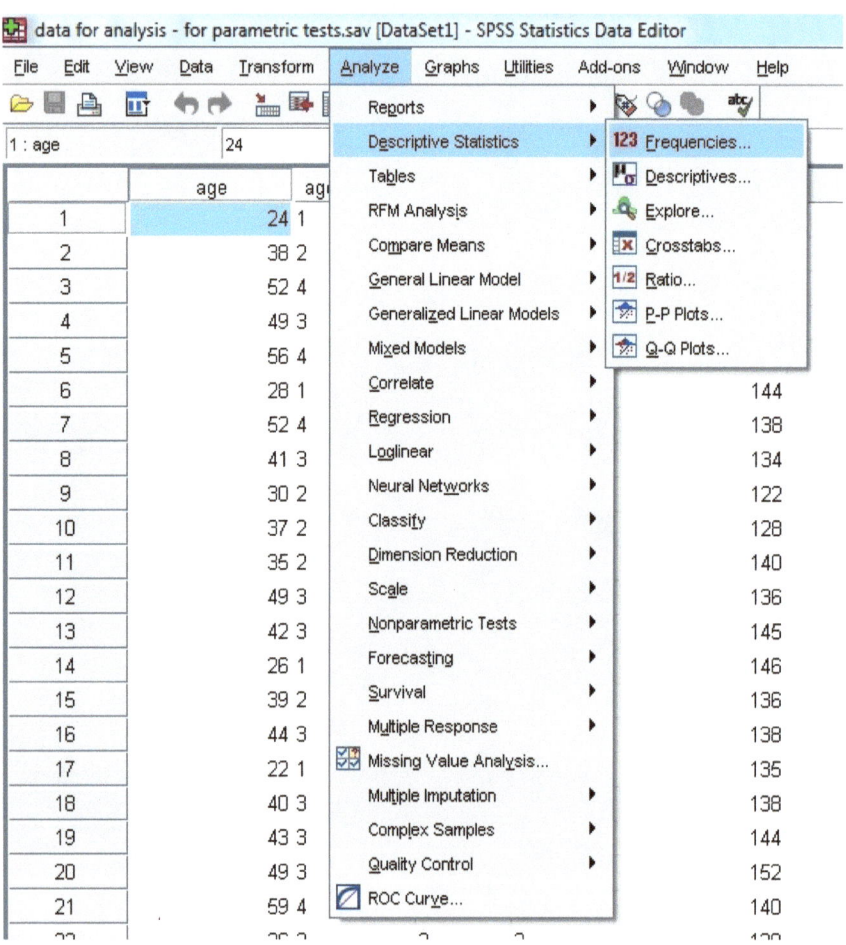

Select the continuous variable to be described

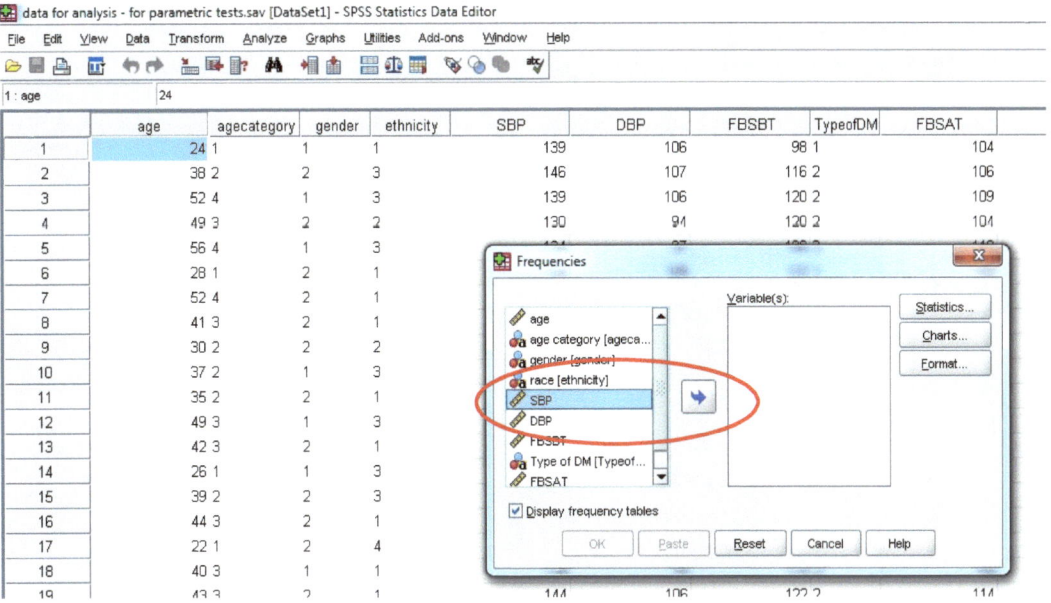

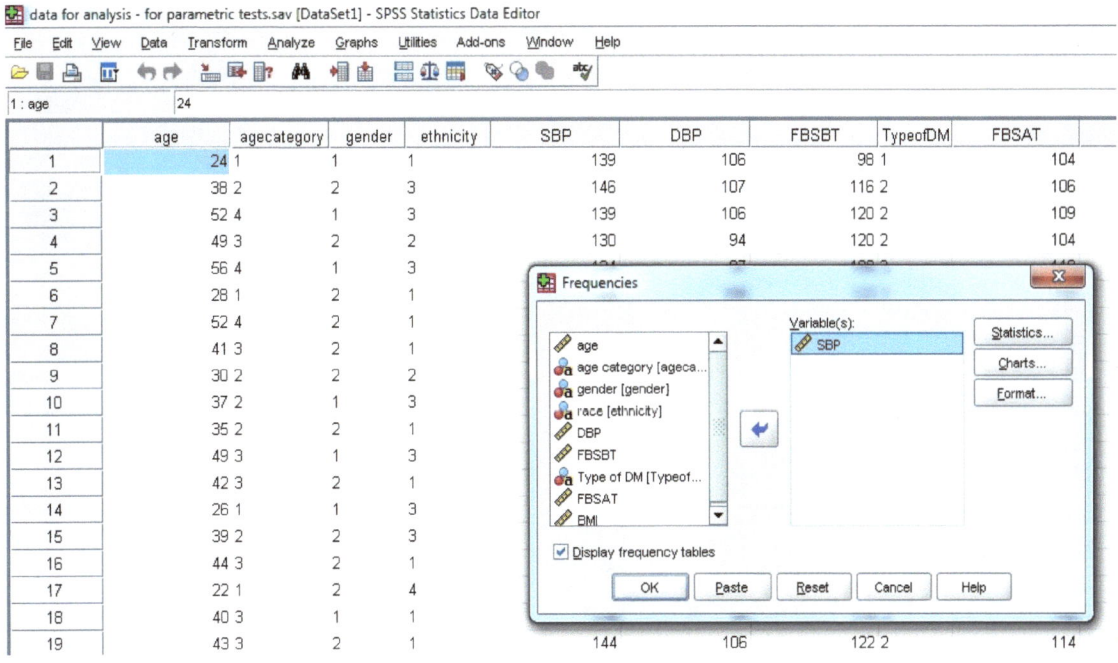

Click Statistics ------- Select the statistics required

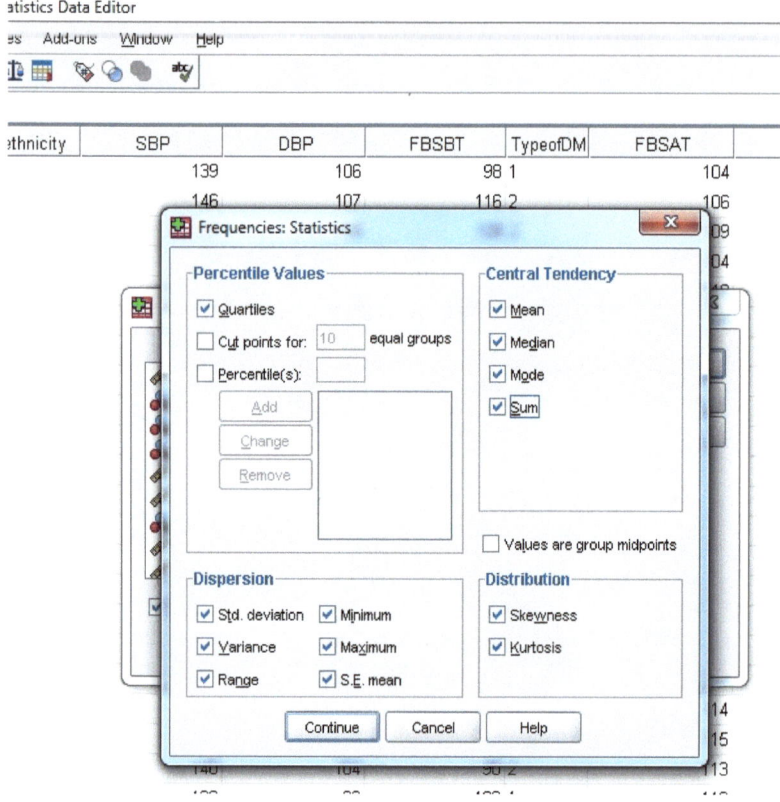

Click continue

Click Charts

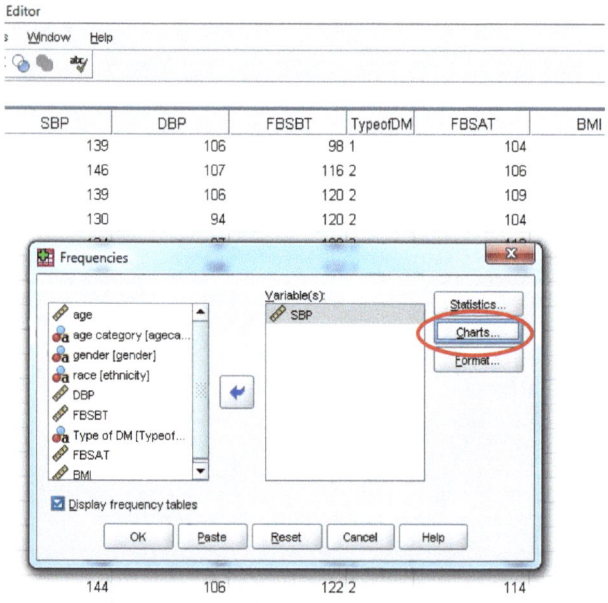

If you want to draw a histogram with normal curve, click Histograms and Tick 'With normal curve'

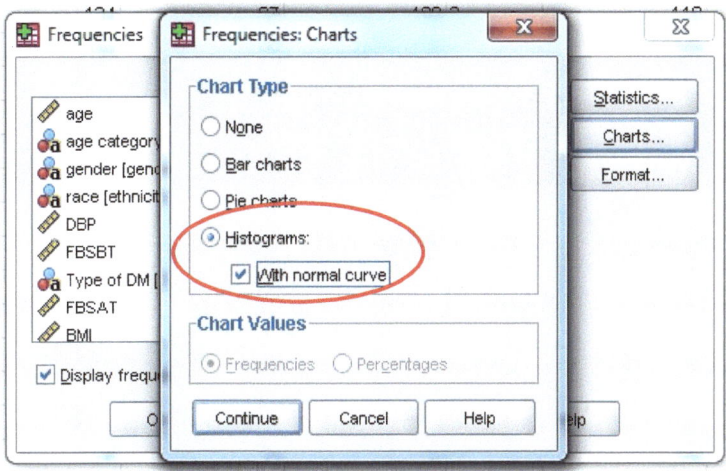

Click continue --------------- then click OK

Result will open as Output1 in SPSS Statistics viewer window.

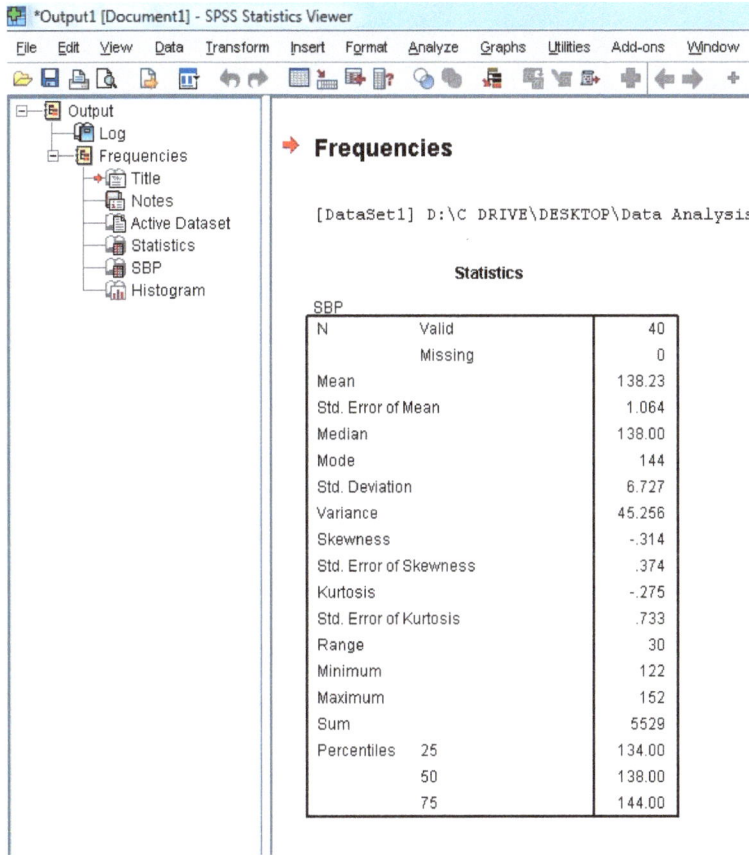

All the requested statistics will be displayed.

Histogram

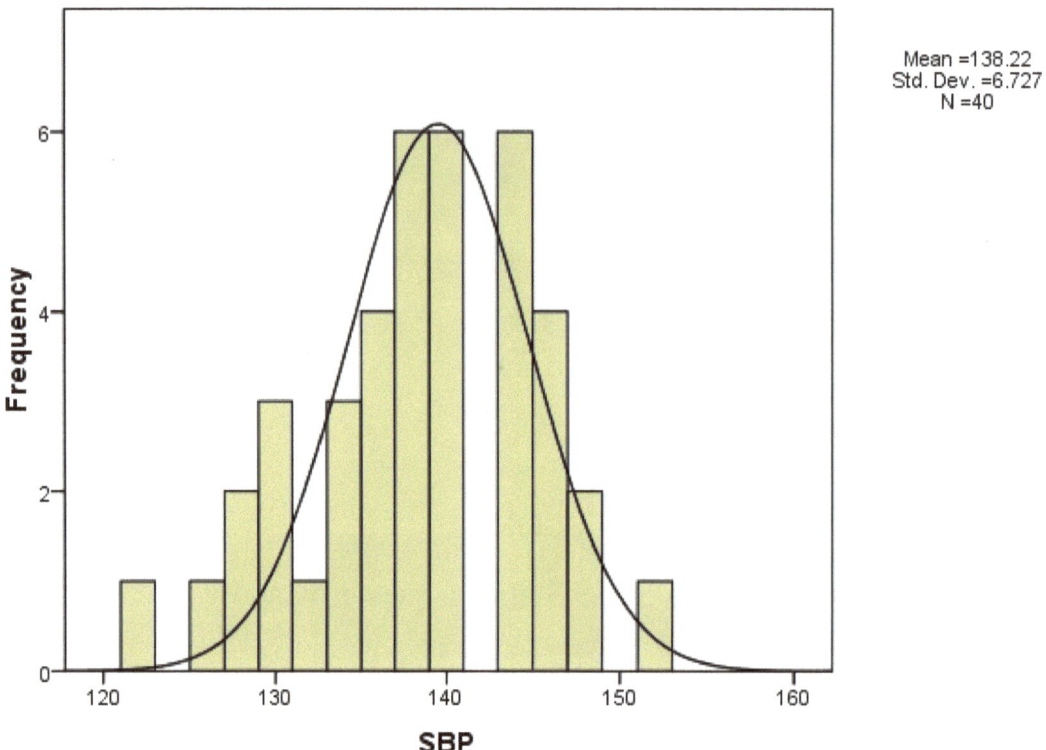

Histogram with normal distribution curve will be displayed. It will be discussed in the following session on Normality of data.

Method 2

For descriptive statistics of continuous variable

Click Analyze ---------- Descriptive Statistics -------------- Explore

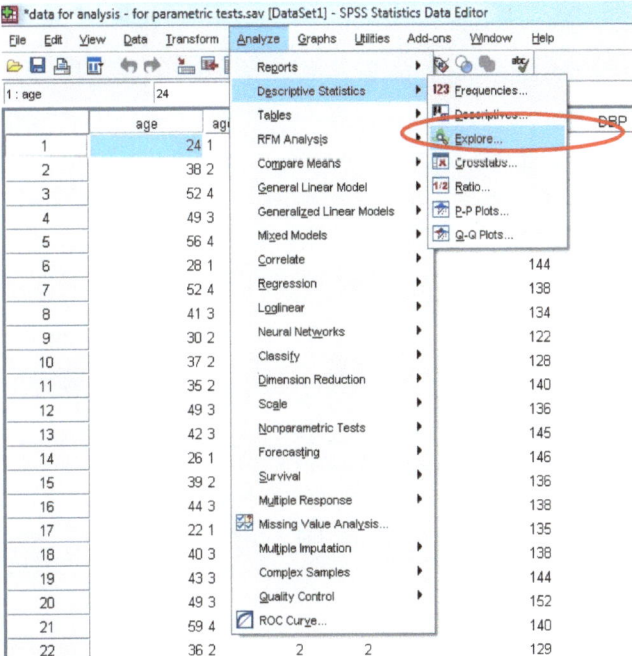

Select the continuous variable to be described

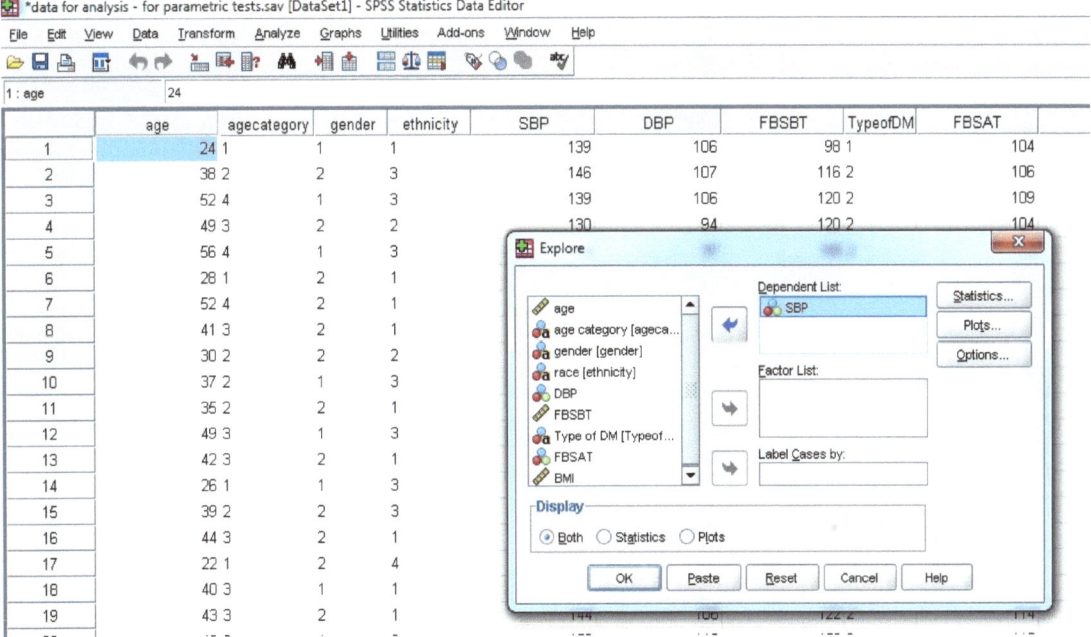

Click Statistics ------- Select the statistics required

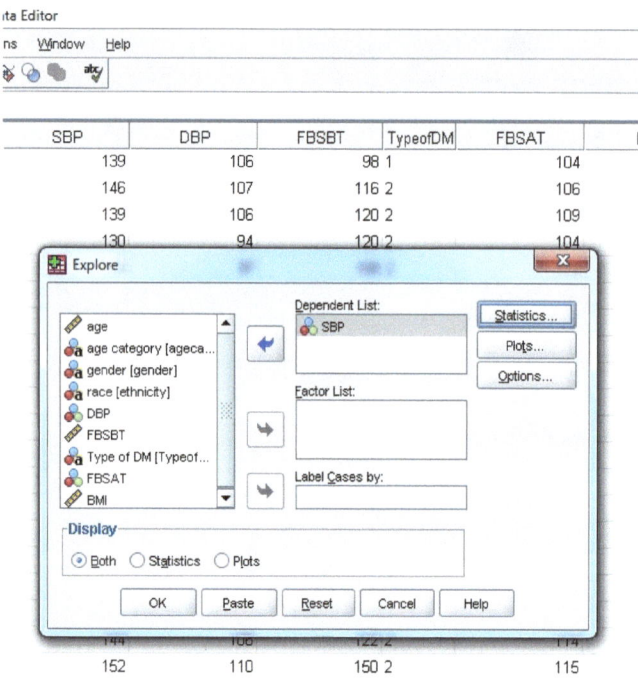

Click Descriptive ----------- Click percentiles and outliers (if want to spot outliers)

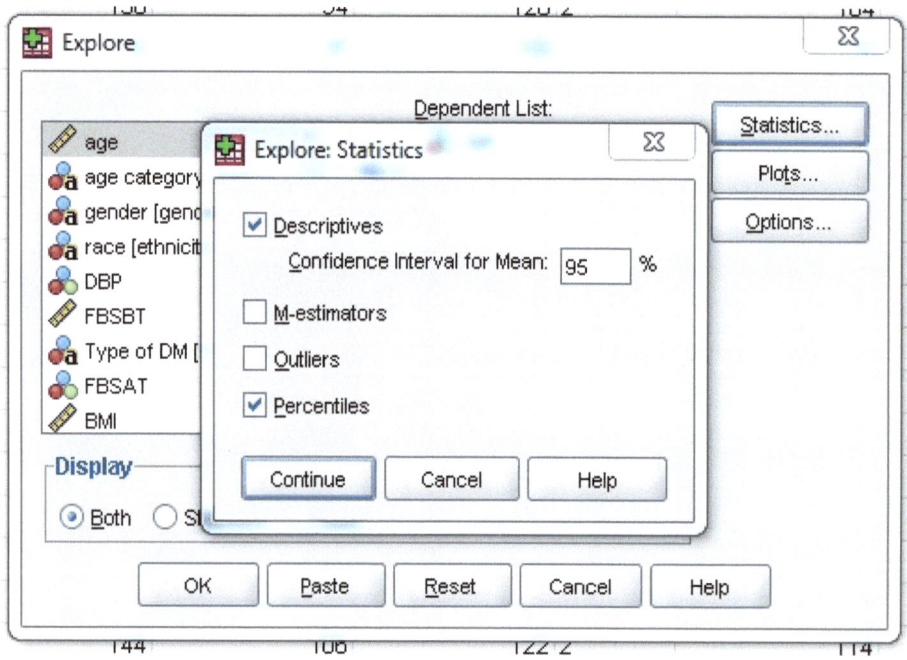

Click continue

Click Plots ------------- Click Stem and Leaf plot or Histogram as required

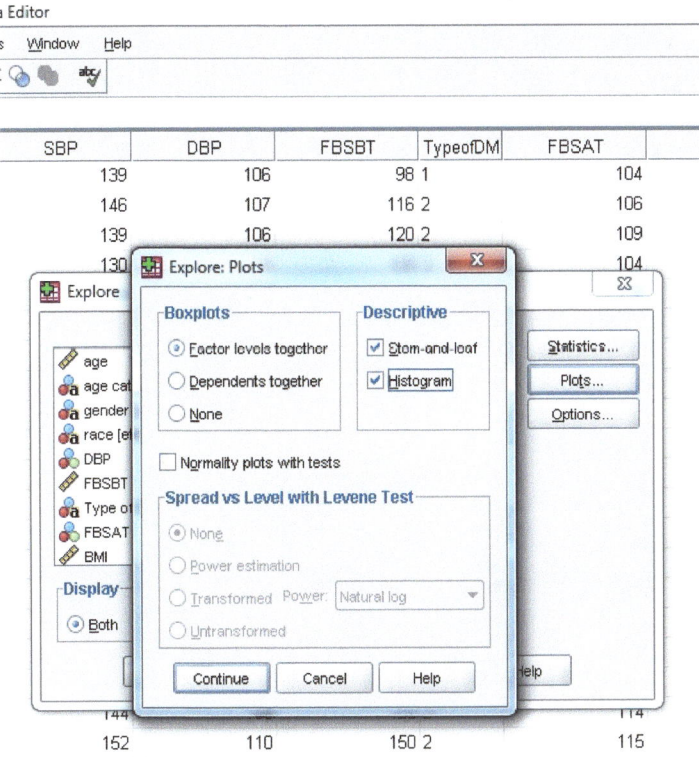

Click Normality plots with tests – to know if the data is normally distributed

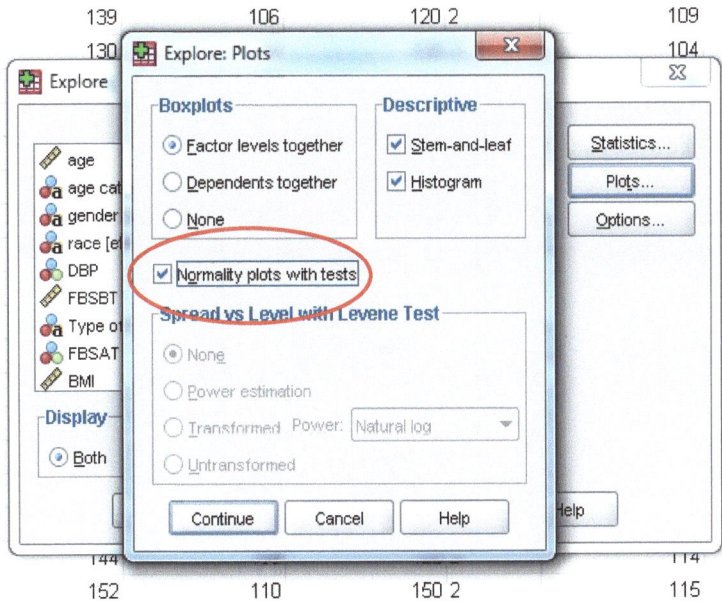

Click continue – then display both Statistics and Plots

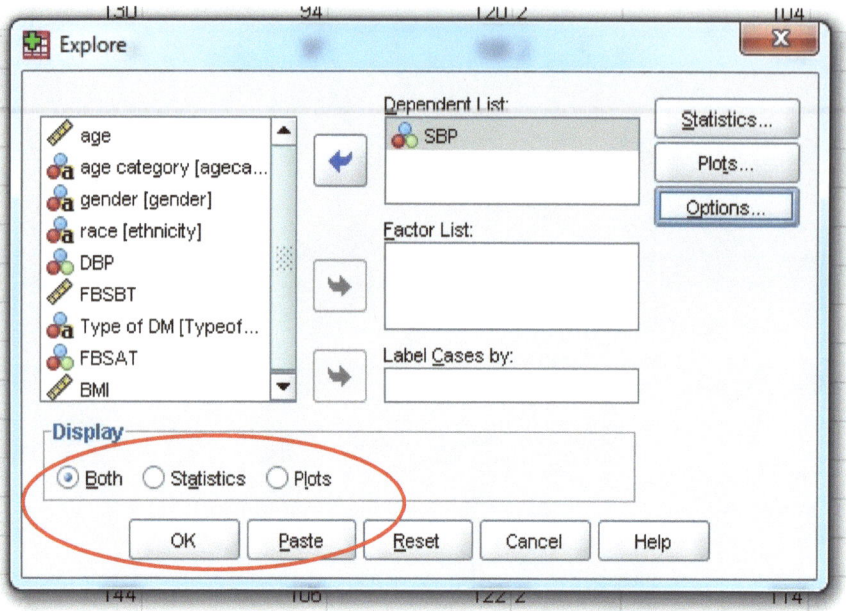

Click OK

Result will open as Output1 in SPSS Statistics viewer window.

Descriptive statistics is as follows

Descriptives

			Statistic	Std. Error
SBP	Mean		138.23	1.064
	95% Confidence Interval for Mean	Lower Bound	136.07	
		Upper Bound	140.38	
	5% Trimmed Mean		138.36	
	Median		138.00	
	Variance		45.256	
	Std. Deviation		6.727	
	Minimum		122	
	Maximum		152	
	Range		30	
	Interquartile Range		10	
	Skewness		-.314	.374
	Kurtosis		-.275	.733

Advantage of this method – Can know the 95% confidence interval values of the continuous variable

Test of Normality table will be displayed.

Test of Normality – Method 1

Shapiro Wilk Test

Tests of Normality

	Kolmogorov-Smirnov[a]			Shapiro-Wilk		
	Statistic	df	Sig.	Statistic	df	Sig.
SBP	.130	40	.088	.977	40	.564

a. Lilliefors Significance Correction

Shapiro Wilk test is chosen because it can be applied even if the sample size is either very low or very big. If Sig. value of Shapiro Wilk test is >0.05, null hypothesis is accepted. Null hypothesis is that data is normally distributed.

In simple terms, if Sig. value is >0.05 for Shapiro Wilk test, the data is normally distributed.

Normality Plots are also shown in the output

Test of Normality – Method 2

Q-Q Plot is used for plotting normality.

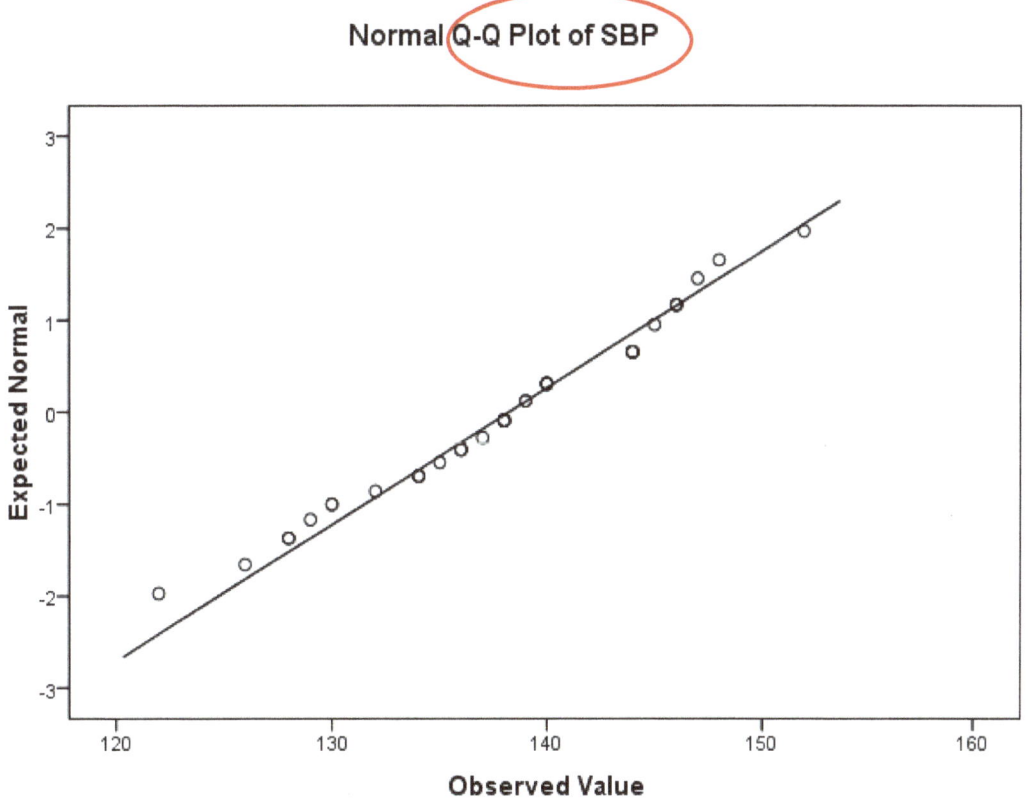

Normal Q-Q Plot of SBP

If the observations are centred around the slope, the data is considered normally distributed. But Q-Q plots shows subjective variations between the observers.

So Shapiro Wilk test is the most preferred method to test the normality.

Test of Normality – Method 3

By looking at the Histogram with Normality curve

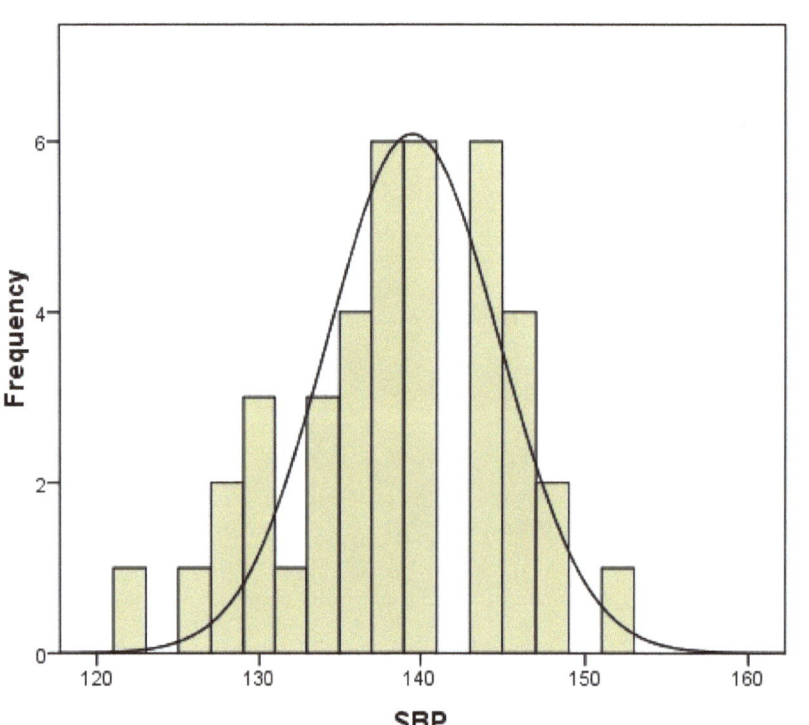

Histogram

Histogram with normal curve shows that the data is normally distributed. But for selection of appropriate test of significance, we need to confirm normality with tests of normality.

Test of Normality – Method 4

By looking at the values of mean, median and mode
If Mean, median and mode are almost same – Data is normally distributed
If Mean and Median are away from mode – Data is skewed towards the side of mean.
If mean is higher than mode – Data is skewed towards right or positively skewed.
If mean is lower than mode – Data is skewed towards left or negatively skewed.

Test of Normality – Method 5

By looking at the Box and Whisker plot

Box and Whisker plot of a normally distributed dataset appears as below

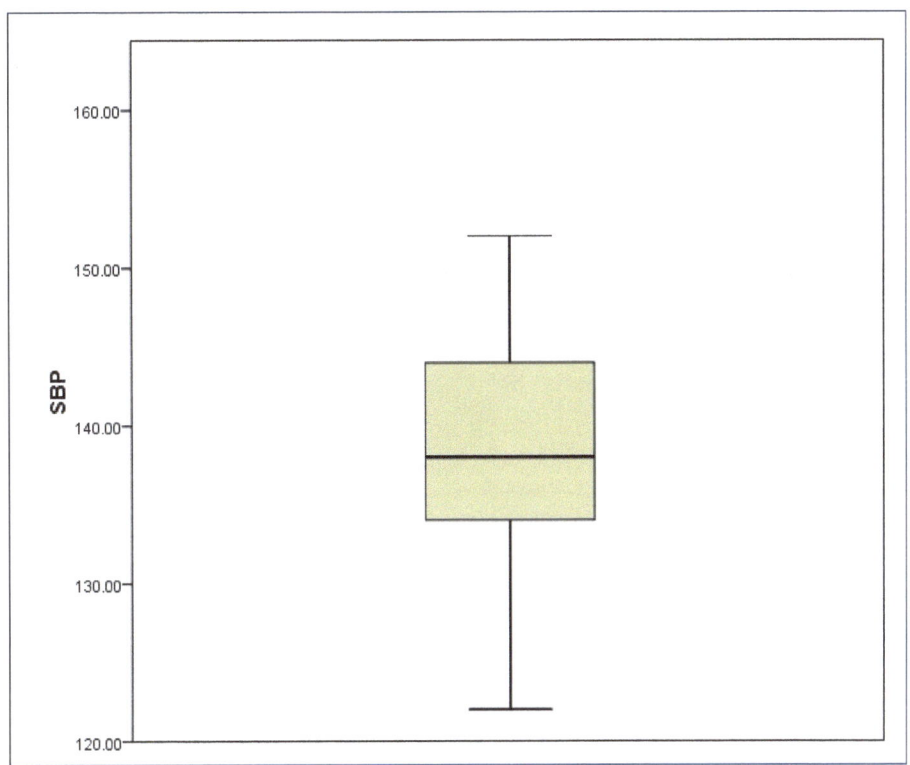

1. Two whiskers will be of almost equal length
2. The transverse line inside the box, which corresponds to median will be approximately at the centre of the box.

Box and Whisker plot of a not normally distributed or skewed dataset appears as below

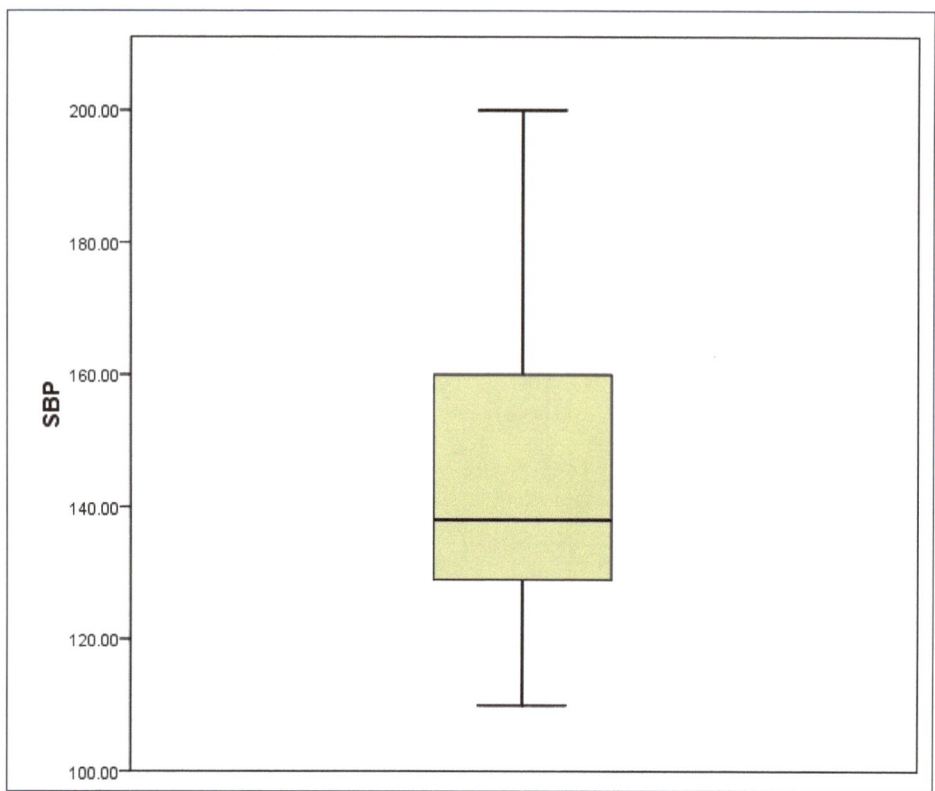

1. Two whiskers will be of un equal length
2. The transverse line inside the box, which corresponds to median will not be at the centre of the box.

Chapter 3

DESCRIPTIVE STATISTICS OF CATEGORICAL VARIABLES USING SPSS

Click Analyze ---------- Descriptive Statistics -------------- Frequencies

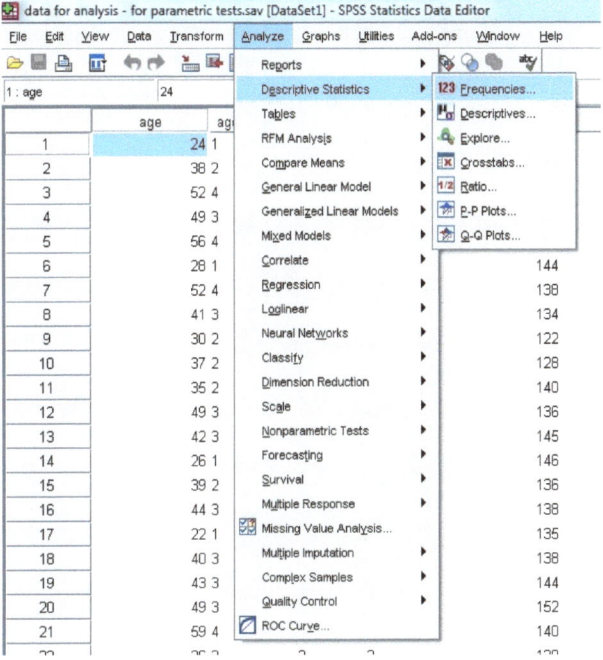

Select the categorical variable to be described

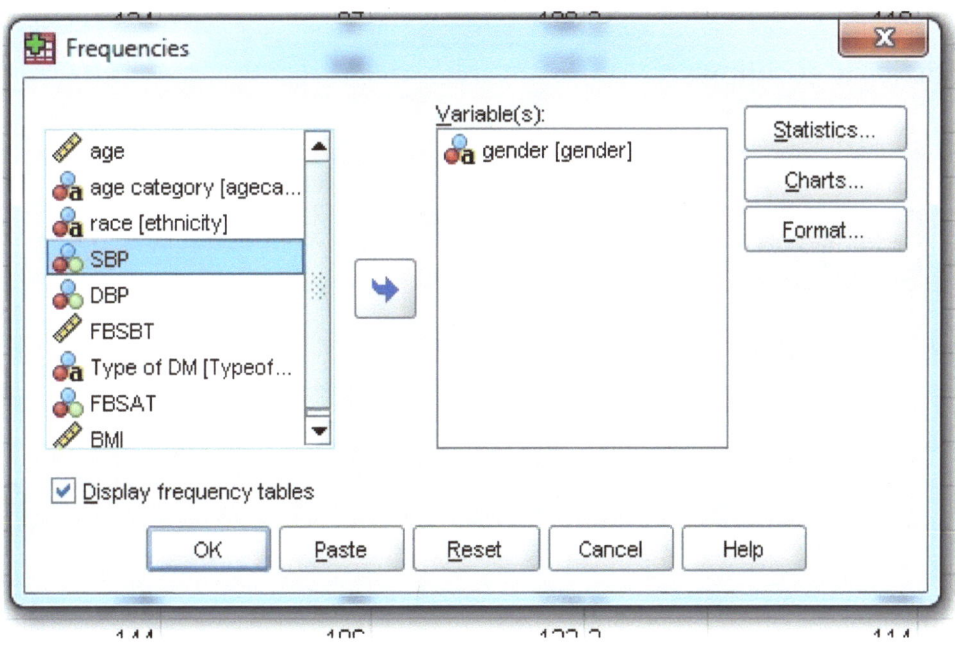

Click Charts

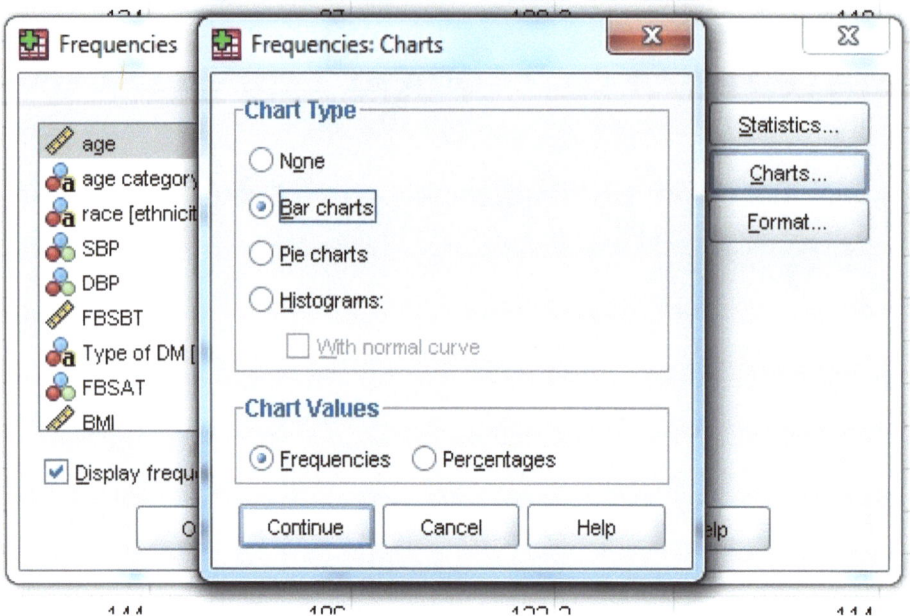

Select either Bar charts or Pie charts as per your requirement

Select chart values as either Frequencies or Percentages

Then click Continue

Then click OK

Result will open as Output1 in SPSS Statistics viewer window.

Descriptive statistics is as follows.

Statistics

gender

N	Valid	40
	Missing	0

gender

		Frequency	Percent	Valid Percent	Cumulative Percent
Valid	male	18	45.0	45.0	45.0
	female	22	55.0	55.0	100.0
	Total	40	100.0	100.0	

Frequency distribution table of the selected categorical variable is displayed

Either Bar diagram or Pie diagram will be displayed as per your request.

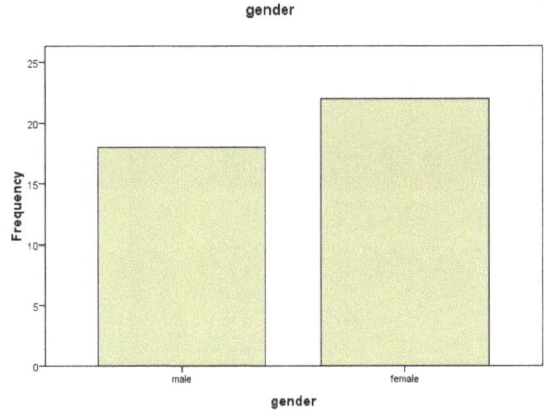

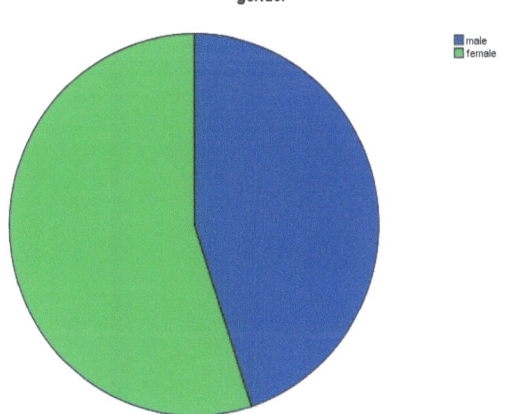

Chapter 4

STUDY OF ASSOCIATION BETWEEN TWO CATEGORICAL VARIABLES - CHI SQUARE TEST USING SPSS

After entering the same data in SPSS data editor

Click Analyze – Descriptive Statistics - Crosstabs

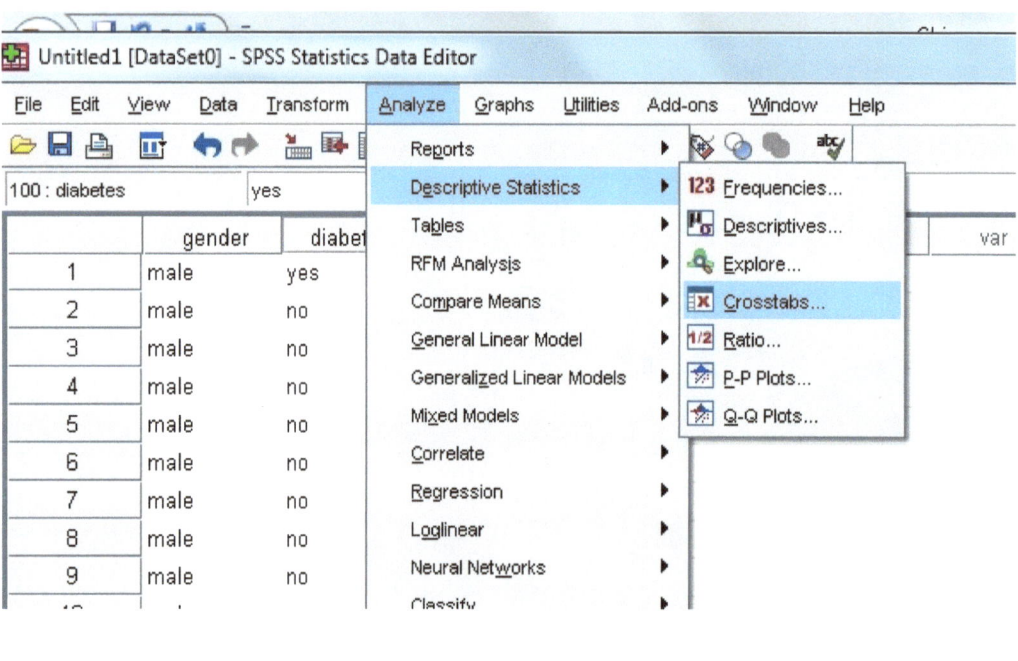

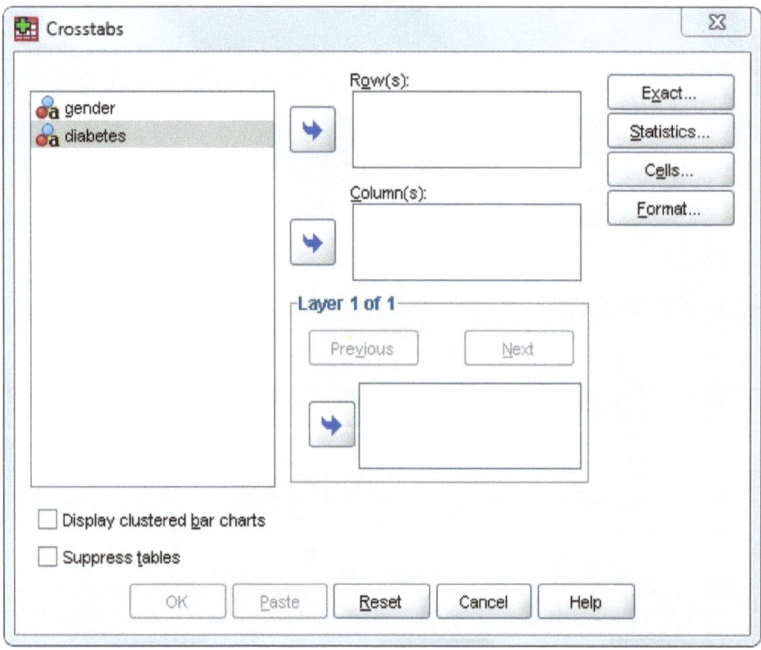

Select 2 categorical variables (eg:- gender and diabetes status) into row and column.

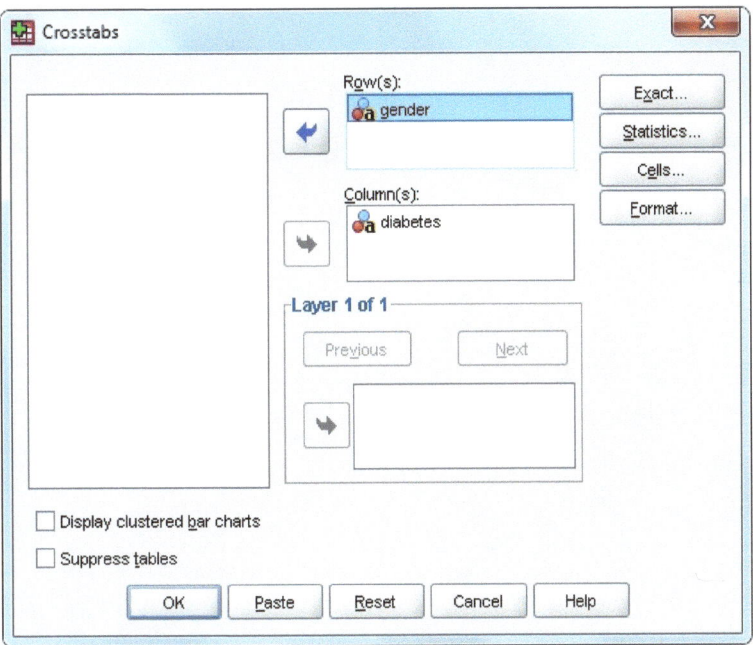

Click statistics – select chi square – click continue

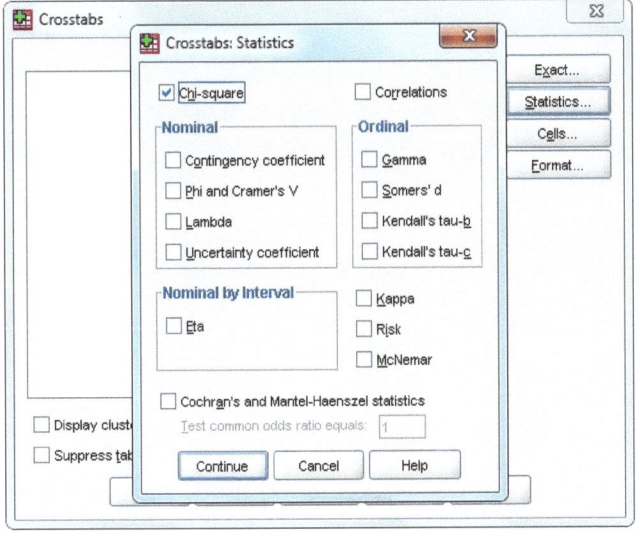

Click cells – Click observed in counts – Click Row, Column and Total percentages – Click continue

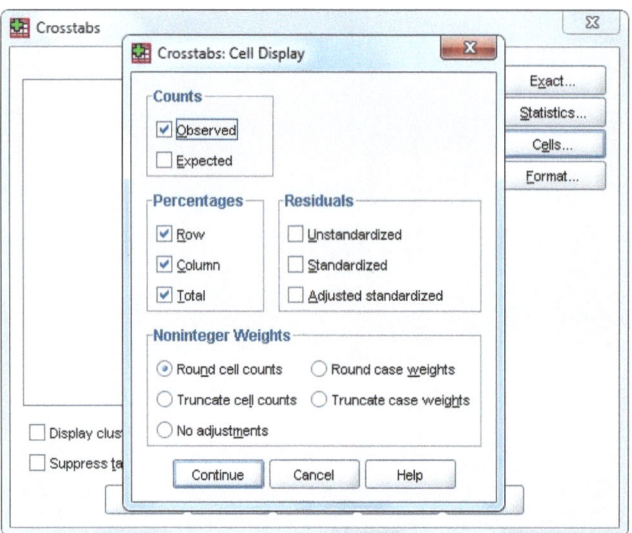

If any of the cells have frequencies less than 5, then click Exact. If all the cells are having more than 5 no. observations, no need for clicking exact.

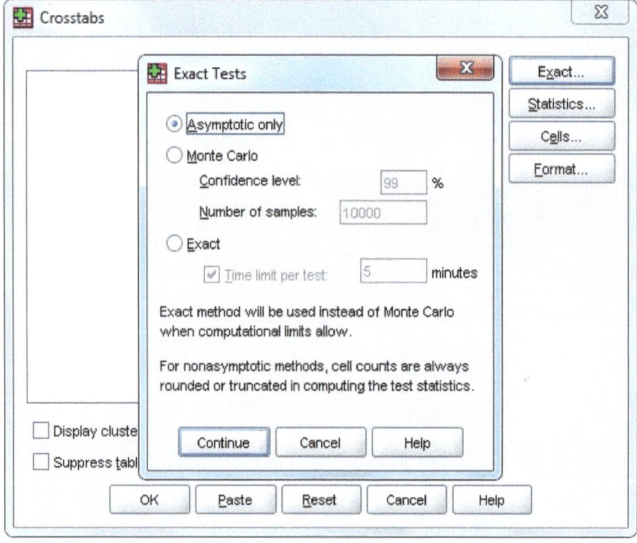

Select Exact – Tick time limit per test 5 minutes – Click continue. For next 5 minutes exact command will be active. After that the command will be shifted from exact to asymptotic significant value.

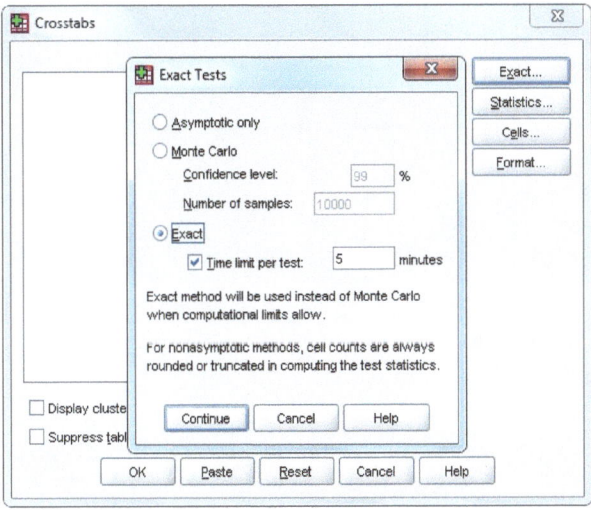

Click Continue and OK

The result of Chi square analysis will be as follows

Case Processing Summary

	Cases					
	Valid		Missing		Total	
	N	Percent	N	Percent	N	Percent
gender * diabetes	100	100.0%	0	.0%	100	100.0%

gender * diabetes Crosstabulation

			diabetes		Total
			no	yes	
gender	female	Count	35	15	50
		% within gender	70.0%	30.0%	100.0%
		% within diabetes	43.8%	75.0%	50.0%
		% of Total	35.0%	15.0%	50.0%
	male	Count	45	5	50
		% within gender	90.0%	10.0%	100.0%
		% within diabetes	56.3%	25.0%	50.0%
		% of Total	45.0%	5.0%	50.0%
Total		Count	80	20	100
		% within gender	80.0%	20.0%	100.0%
		% within diabetes	100.0%	100.0%	100.0%
		% of Total	80.0%	20.0%	100.0%

Shows the count and percentages in each groups of categorical variables

Chi-Square Tests

	Value	df	Asymp. Sig. (2-sided)	Exact Sig. (2 sided)	Exact Sig. (1 sided)
Pearson Chi-Square	6.250[a]	1	.012		
Continuity Correction[b]	5.063	1	.024		
Likelihood Ratio	6.486	1	.011		
Fisher's Exact Test				.023	.011
N of Valid Cases	100				

a. 0 cells (.0%) have expected count less than 5. The minimum expected count is 10.00.

b. Computed only for a 2x2 table

Pearson Chi square value is 6.25 and degree of freedom (df) is 1. Asymp. Sig means Asymptotic significance value and is the p value. Here the Asymp. Sig value is <0.05, the difference in occurrence of outcome in different groups is statistically significant.

If Asymp. Sig value is ≥0.05, the difference is not statistically significant.

If any of the cells in the table is having expected value less than 5, exact significance value should be chosen.

Interpretation of findings

Here the prevalence of diabetes among females is significantly higher than the prevalence of diabetes among males.

Chapter 5

COMPARISON BETWEEN TWO OR MORE MEANS

When data is normally distributed – Apply parametric tests of significance

When data is not normally distributed / skewed – Apply non – parametric tests of significance

Parametric tests for continuous data	Equivalent Non – parametric tests for continuous data
1 sample T test	Mann Whitney U test / Wilcoxon Signed Rank test
Paired T test	Mann Whitney U test / Wilcoxon Signed Rank test
2 sample T test	Mann Whitney U test / Wilcoxon Signed Rank test
ANOVA test	Kruskal Wallis test

1 sample T test

Used to compare the mean value of a continuous variable with a standard value or reference value. Reference value is obtained from guidelines or standard text book or previous research.

It is a parametric test, which is applied when data is normally distributed

2 sample T test or Independent samples T test

2 sample T test – is applied to test if the difference in mean values of a continuous variable between 2 different groups is statistically significant. Eg: Comparison between mean blood sugar values of male patients and mean blood sugar values of female patients.

One variable is a continuous variable (Eg:- blood sugar values). The other variable is a categorical variable with 2 categories (Eg:- gender, family history of diabetes, etc)

It is a parametric test, which is applied when data is normally distributed

Paired T test

Paired T test – is applied to test if the difference in mean values in the same sample at 2 different times is statistically significant. Eg: comparison of mean haemoglobin values of a group of patients before and after treatment.

It is a parametric test, which is applied when data is normally distributed

Wilcoxon Signed Rank test / Mann Whitney U test is applied to test if the difference between continuous variables between 2 groups of individuals is statistically significant. Sample size of both groups should be same. It is a non – parametric test of significance and can be applied for either paired sample or independent samples.

It is applied when either of the two continuous dataset is not normally distributed

ANOVA test (Analysis of Variance) – is applied to test if the difference in mean values of a continuous variable between more than 2 different groups is statistically significant.

Eg: Hb values of patients of different ethnic origin (malay, Chinese, indian and others).

It's a parametric test – applied to normally distributed data.

One variable is a continuous variable (eg:- hemoglobin values, blood sugar values, BMI etc.)

Other variable is a categorical variable having more than 2 categories (Eg:- ethnicity, education level, occupation, etc).

Kruskal Wallis test - is a non-parametric test of significance for testing if the difference between more than two independent groups are statistically significant.

It is a non-parametric test of significance and an alternative to ANOVA test, which can be applied when data is not normally distributed.

One variable is a continuous variable (eg:- hemoglobin values, blood sugar values, BMI etc.)

Other variable is a categorical variable having more than 2 categories (Eg:- ethnicity, education level, occupation, etc).

How to do One Sample T test

It is a parametric test, which is applied when data is normally distributed and is done to compare the mean value of a continuous variable with a standard value or reference value.

Analyze ---------- Compare means-------------------- One sample T test

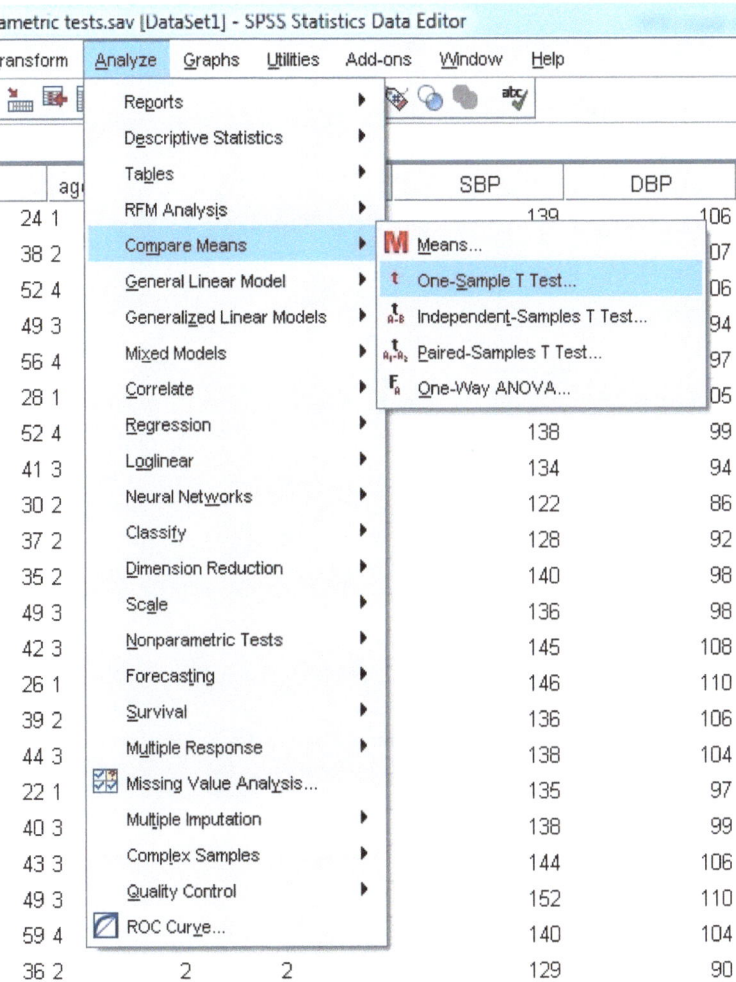

Then the following window appears

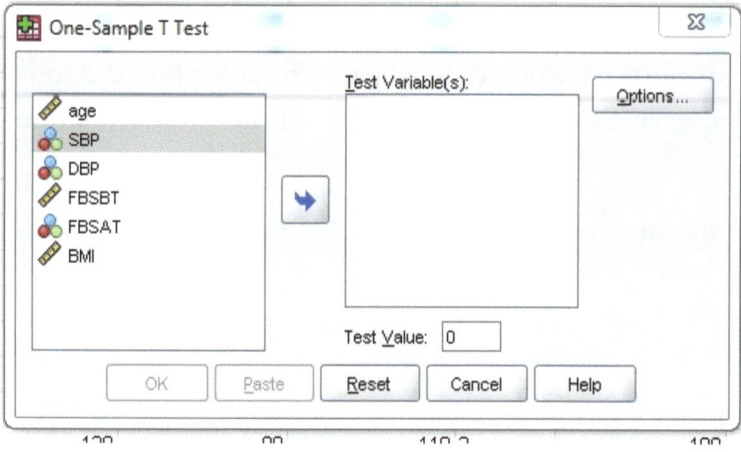

Then select test variable and test value.

For example, here we can select SBP (Systolic Blood pressure) as the test variable and 120 mm Hg as the test value

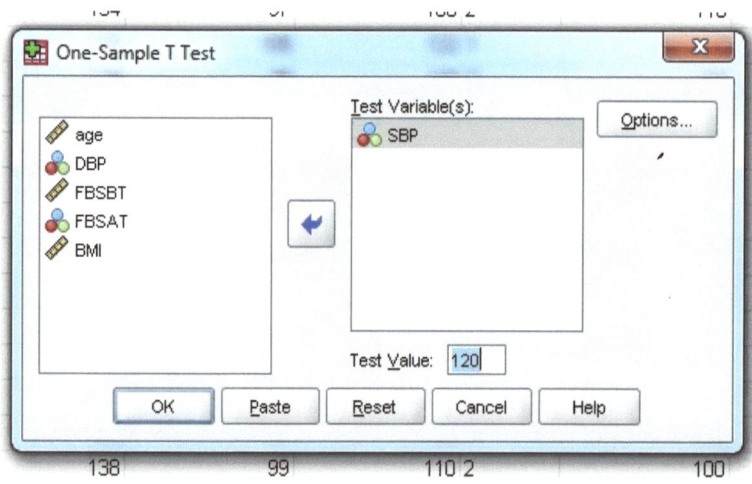

Then click Options

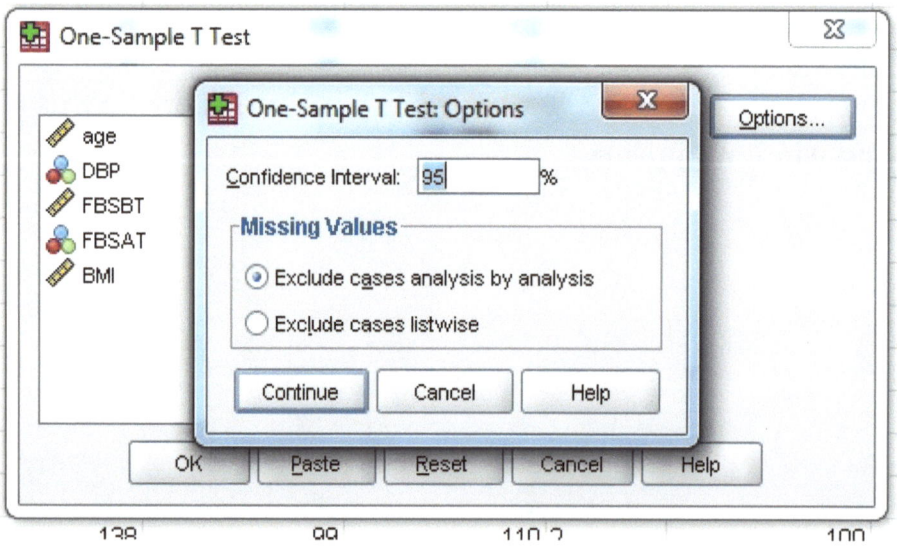

Select 95% confidence intervals

Click continue ----------------- Then click OK

The results appears in Output window as follows

One-Sample Statistics

	N	Mean	Std. Deviation	Std. Error Mean
SBP	40	138.23	6.727	1.064

One-Sample Test

	Test Value = 120					
					95% Confidence Interval of the Difference	
	t	df	Sig. (2-tailed)	Mean Difference	Lower	Upper
SBP	17.134	39	.000	18.225	16.07	20.38

The first table shows the description of test variable.

The second table shows t value, degree of freedom (sample size – 1) and Sig. value (P value).

2 tailed sig. value means that the difference of mean value of test variable can be either lower or higher than the test value. This is same as 2 sided distribution.

Interpretation 1 - Here the mean SBP value is significantly different from the test value of 120 mm Hg. (Sig. value is < 0.05).

Difference between mean SBP value in the sample and the test value is 18.225 and the 95% confidence interval of difference between means is between 16.07 and 20.38.

Interpretation 2 - If the study is repeated 100 times, 95% of times, the difference between mean SBP and the test value will be between 16.07 and 20.38. Since the range of 95% confidence interval of difference is not including zero, the difference between mean SBP value and the test value is statistically significant.

How to do Independent Samples T test (2 Samples T test)

Independent samples T test – is applied to test if the difference in mean values of a continuous variable between 2 different groups is statistically significant.

One variable is a continuous variable. The other variable is a categorical variable with 2 categories (Eg:- gender, disease status or any dichotomous variable)

Analyze ------- Compare means------- Independent Samples T test

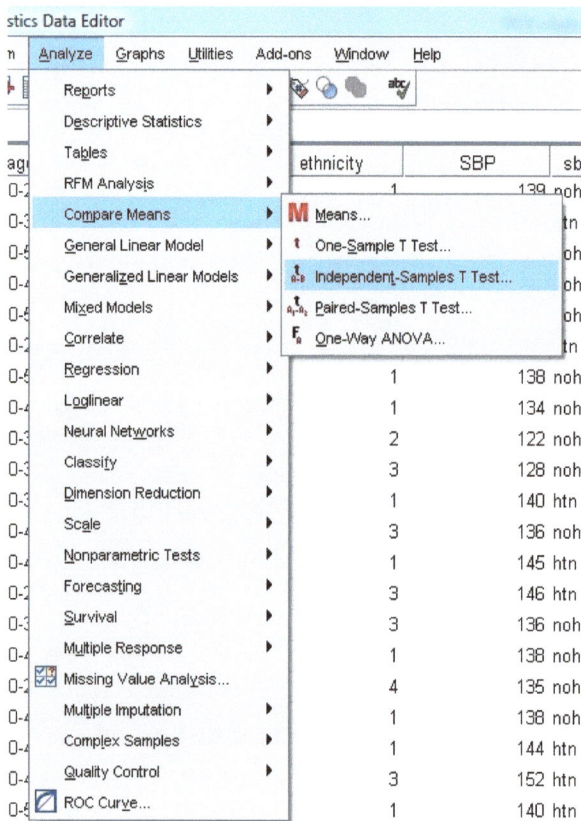

Then the following window appears

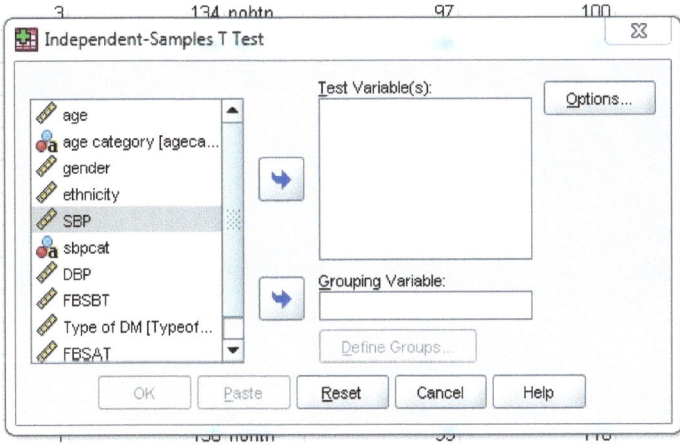

Then select test variable (continuous variable) and the grouping variable (dichotomous categorical variable. Categorical variable should have only 2 categories. Before analysis, grouping variable must be coded as 1 and 2. (EG:- if gender is the grouping variable, code it as 1 for male and 2 for female.

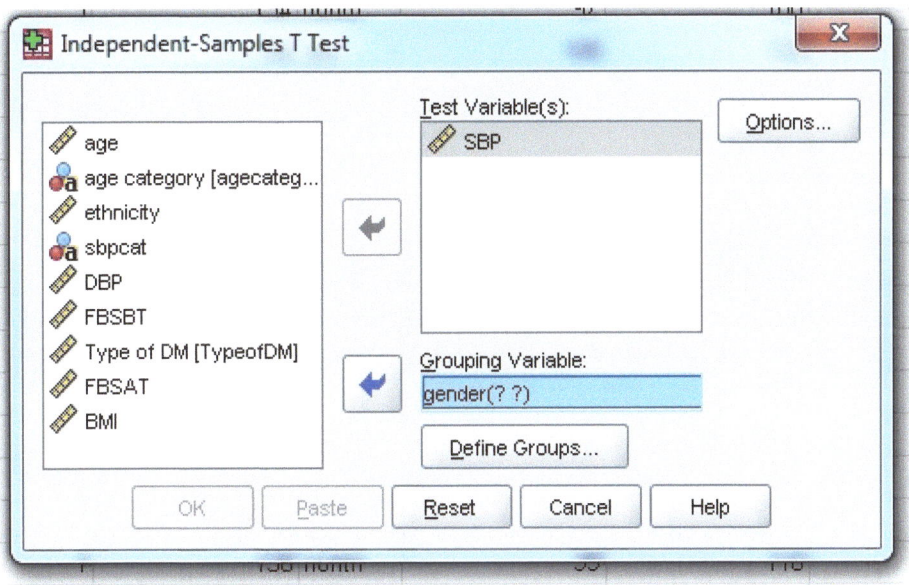

Then click Define Groups

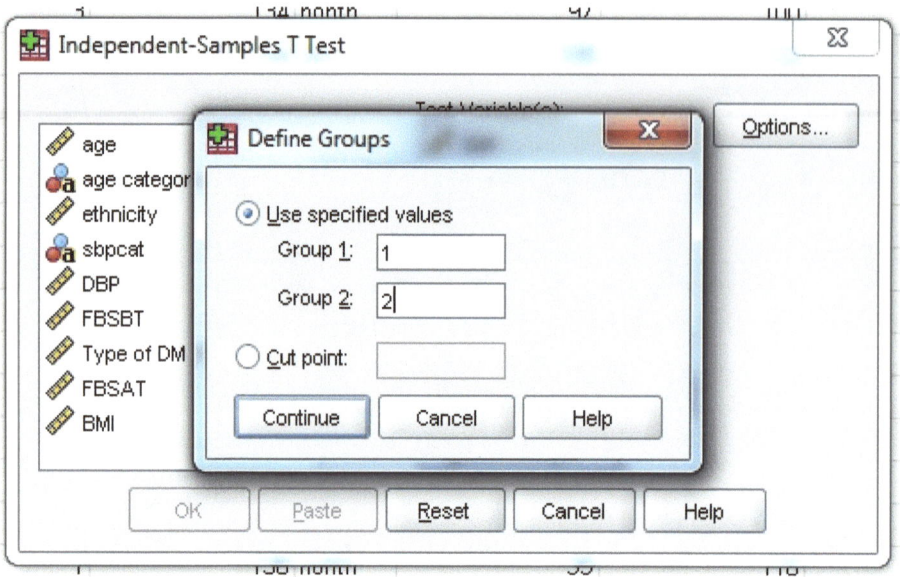

Use specified values 1 for Group 1 (male in this example) and 2 for Group 2 (female in this example).

Then click Continue

Then click Options

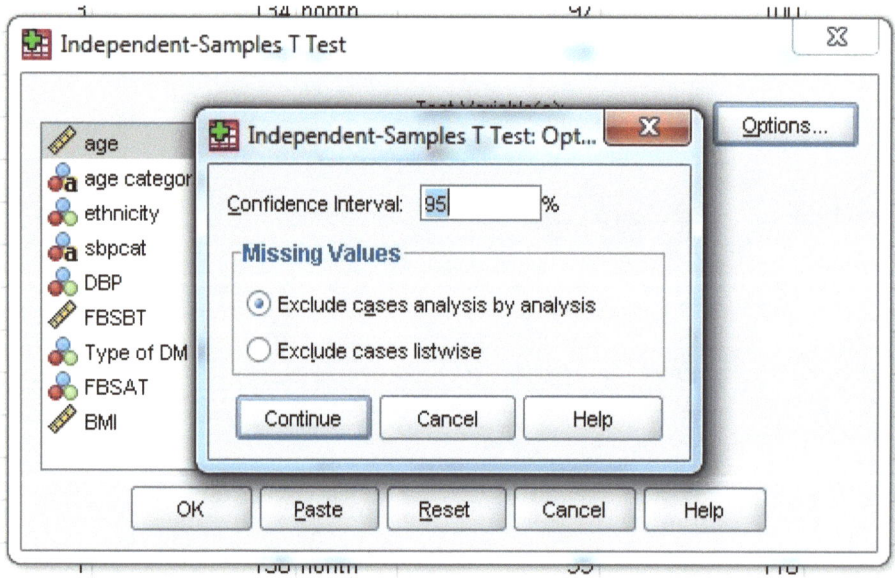

Select 95% confidence intervals

Click continue ----------------- Then click OK

The results appears in Output window as follows

Group Statistics

	gender	N	Mean	Std. Deviation	Std. Error Mean
SBP	1	18	139.44	5.893	1.389
	2	22	137.23	7.322	1.561

Independent Samples Test

		Levene's Test for Equality of Variances		t-test for Equality of Means					95% Confidence Interval of the Difference	
		F	Sig.	t	df	Sig. (2-tailed)	Mean Difference	Std. Error Difference	Lower	Upper
SBP	Equal variances assumed	1.512	.226	1.038	38	.306	2.217	2.136	-2.107	6.541
	Equal variances not assumed			1.061	37.995	.295	2.217	2.090	-2.013	6.447

The first table shows the description of test variable in different categories.

The second table shows t value, degree of freedom $[(n_1+n_2) - 2]$ and Sig. value (P value).

2 tailed sig. value means that the difference of mean value of test variable in group 1 can be either lower or higher than the mean value of test variable in group 2.

If Levene's Test for equality of variances show a significance of <0.05, check for the row with Equal variances assumed. If Levene's Test for equality of variances show a significance of >0.05, check for the row with Equal variances not assumed.

Interpretation 1 – Look for Sig. value (2 tailed) for t-test. If it is <0.05, the difference between means in 2 groups is statistically significant. Here the Sig. value for t test is >0.05. So the difference between means in 2 groups is not statistically significant.

Interpretation 2 - Difference between mean SBP values in group 1 and group 2 is 2.217 and the 95% confidence interval of difference between means in 2 groups is between -2.107 and 6.541 when the equal variances assumed. 95% confidence interval of difference between means in 2 groups is between -2.013 and 6.447 when the equal variances not assumed.

If the study is repeated 100 times, 95% of times, the difference between mean SBP and the test value will be between -2.013 and 6.447 (Levene's test of equality of variance is not significance in the given example. So the second row is chosen which is for equal variance not assumed.)

Since the range of 95% confidence interval of difference is including zero, the difference between mean SBP value among the 2 groups is not statistically significant.

How to do Paired T test

Paired T test – is applied to test if the difference in mean values in the same sample at 2 different times is statistically significant. It is a parametric test, which is applied when data is normally distributed. Paired T test can be used to compare means of 2 related samples.

Analyze ---------- Compare means------------Paired Samples T test

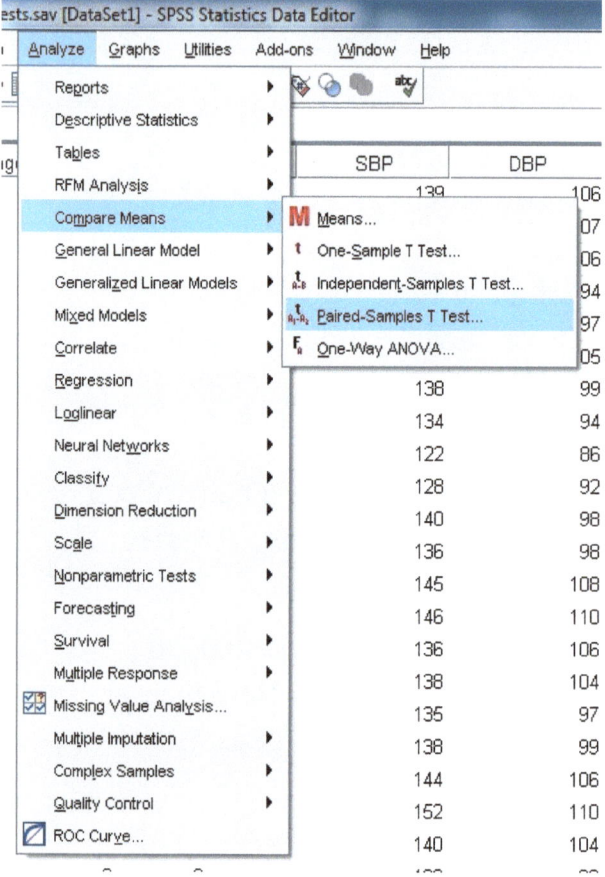

Then the following window appears

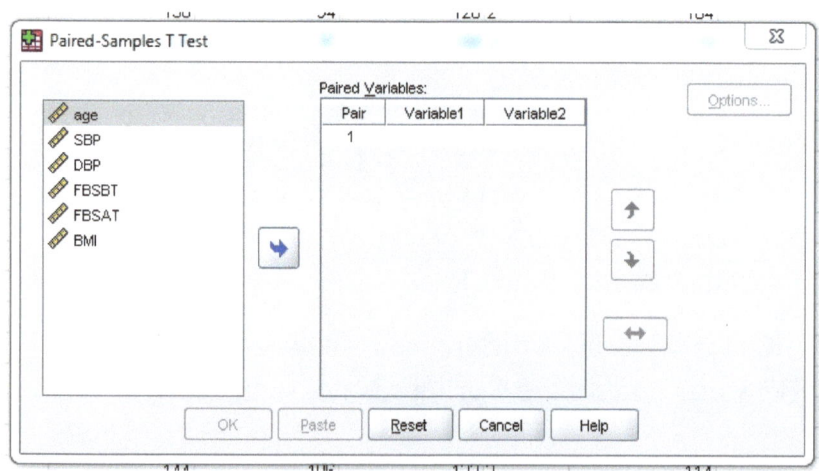

Then select paired variables and move to the analysis window as variable1 and variable2.

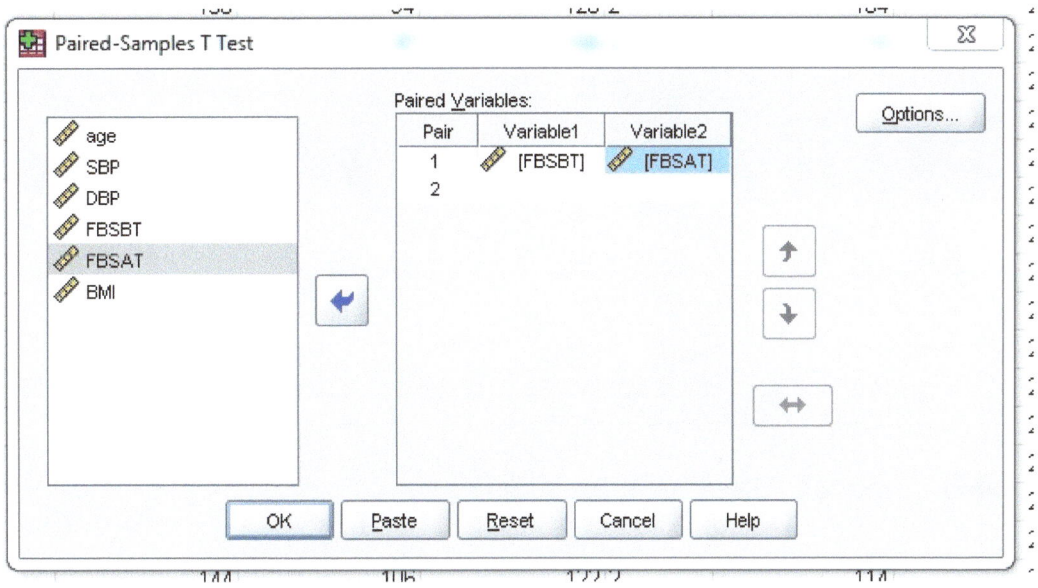

Then click Options --------------------Select 95% confidence interval

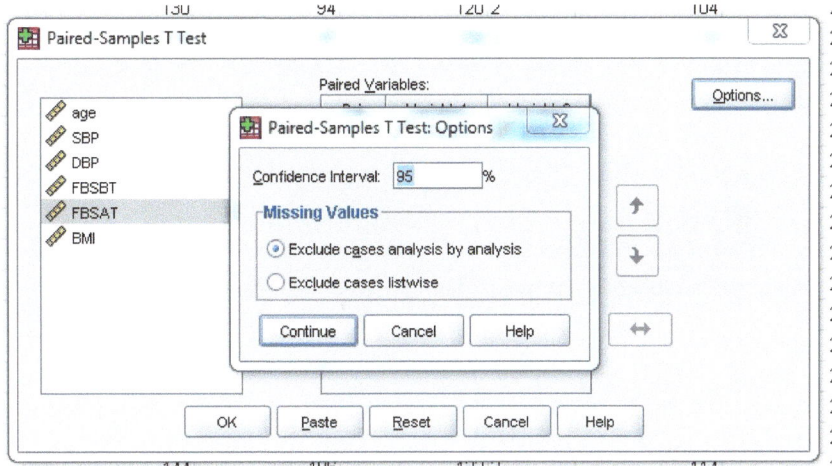

Then click Continue -------------------------------Then OK

The results appears in Output window as follows.

FBSBT and FBSAT are fasting blood sugar values before treatment and fasting blood sugar values after treatment.

Paired Samples Statistics

		Mean	N	Std. Deviation	Std. Error Mean
Pair 1	FBSBT	120.28	40	17.529	2.772
	FBSAT	109.93	40	4.927	.779

Paired Samples Correlations

		N	Correlation	Sig.
Pair 1	FBSBT & FBSAT	40	.407	.009

Paired Samples Test

		Paired Differences							
					95% Confidence Interval of the Difference				
		Mean	Std. Deviation	Std. Error Mean	Lower	Upper	t	df	Sig. (2-tailed)
Pair 1	FBSBT - FBSAT	10.350	16.162	2.555	5.181	15.519	4.050	39	.000

The first table shows the Paired Sample statistics.

The second table shows the correlation between the paired samples. A positive correlation coefficient means that there is a positive correlation between the continuous variables in the paired samples. If Sig. value is less than 0.05, the correlation between the paired samples is statistically significant.

Third table shows difference between means, 95% confidence interval of the difference between mean values, t statistics, degree of freedom (sample size – 1) and Sig. value (P value).

Interpretation 1 – Look for Sig. value (2 tailed) for t-test. If it is <0.05, the difference between means in 2 groups is statistically significant.

Interpretation 2 - Difference between mean FBS values before treatment and after treatment is 10.350 and the 95% confidence interval of difference between means in 2 groups is between 5.181 and 15.519.

If the study is repeated 100 times, 95% of times, the difference between mean FBS values before and after treatment will be between 5.181 and 15.519.

Since the range of 95% confidence interval of difference is not including zero, the difference between mean FBS values before and after treatment is statistically significant.

One way ANOVA test (Analysis of Variance) – is applied to test if the difference in mean values of a continuous variable between more than 2 different groups is statistically significant. It is a parametric test, which is applied when the data is normally distributed.

One variable is a continuous variable and the other variable is a categorical variable having more than 2 categories.

How to do One way ANOVA test

Analyze ---------- Compare means----------- One Way ANOVA

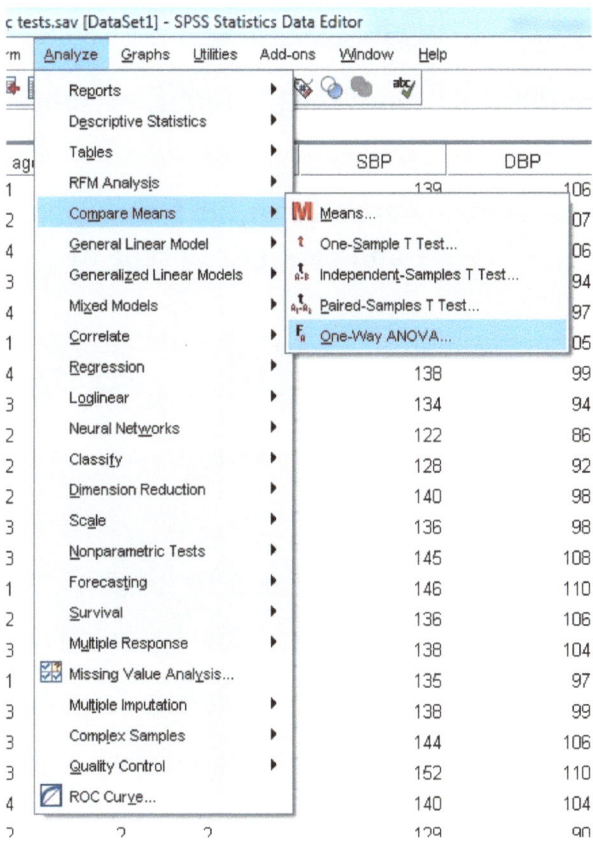

Then the following window appears

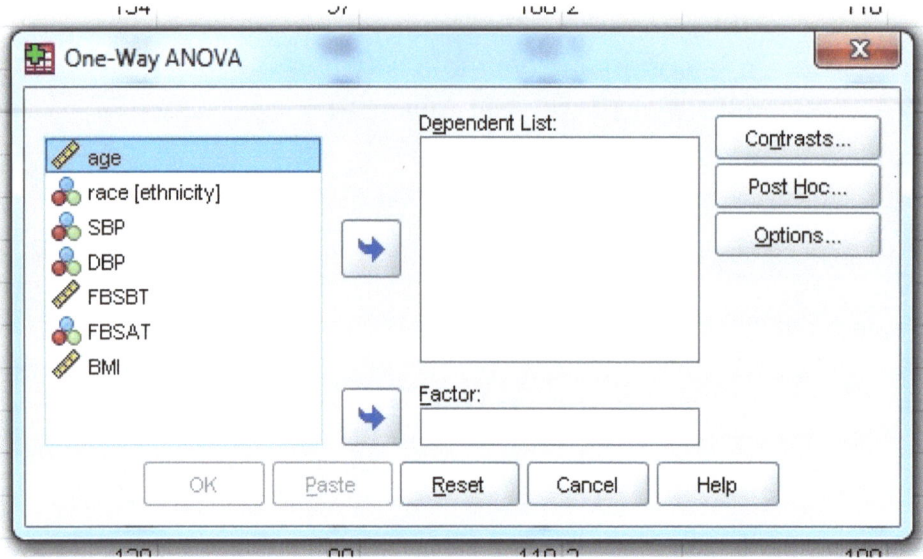

Select the continuous variable as Dependent List and the grouping variable or categorical variable as Factor.

Both Continuous variable and grouping variable must be of the type numeric variables. If not, go to the variable view and change the type of variable as numeric.

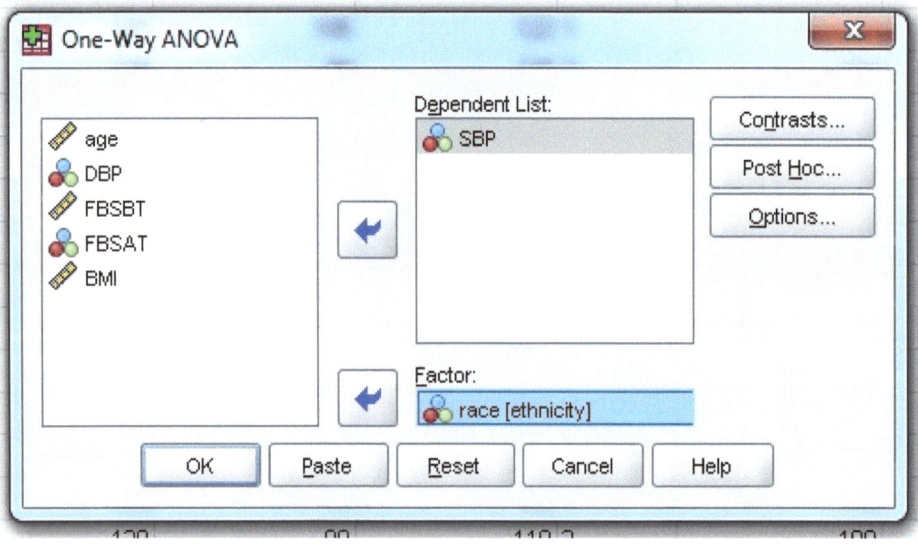

Then click Post Hoc ----------- Post Hoc Multiple Comparisons Window opens

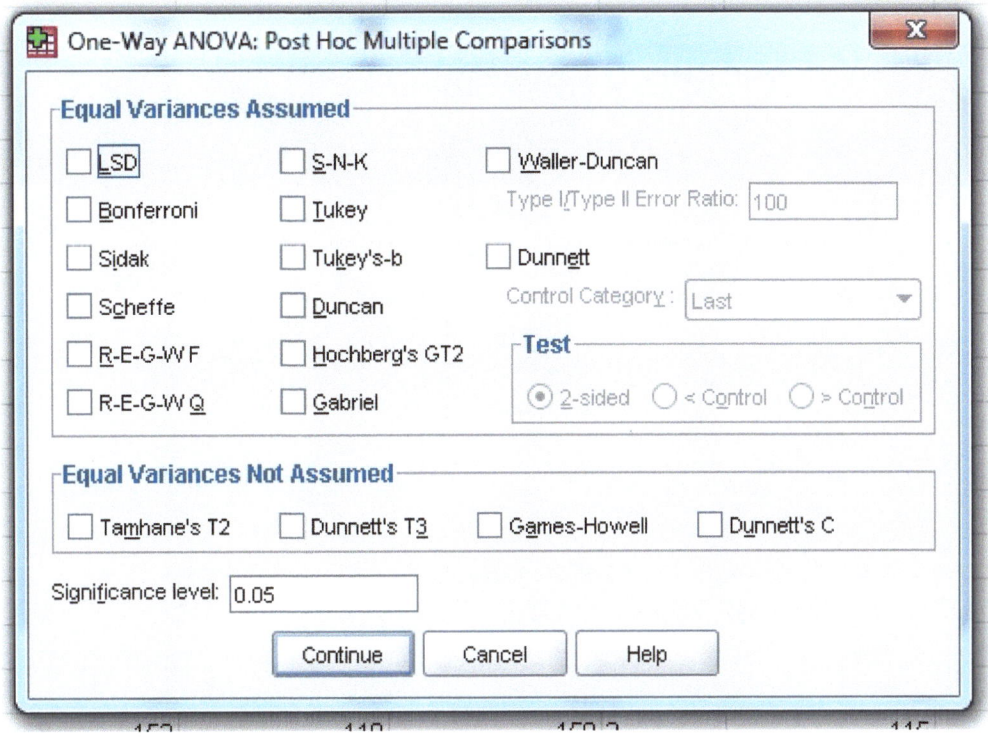

Select Tukey checkbox

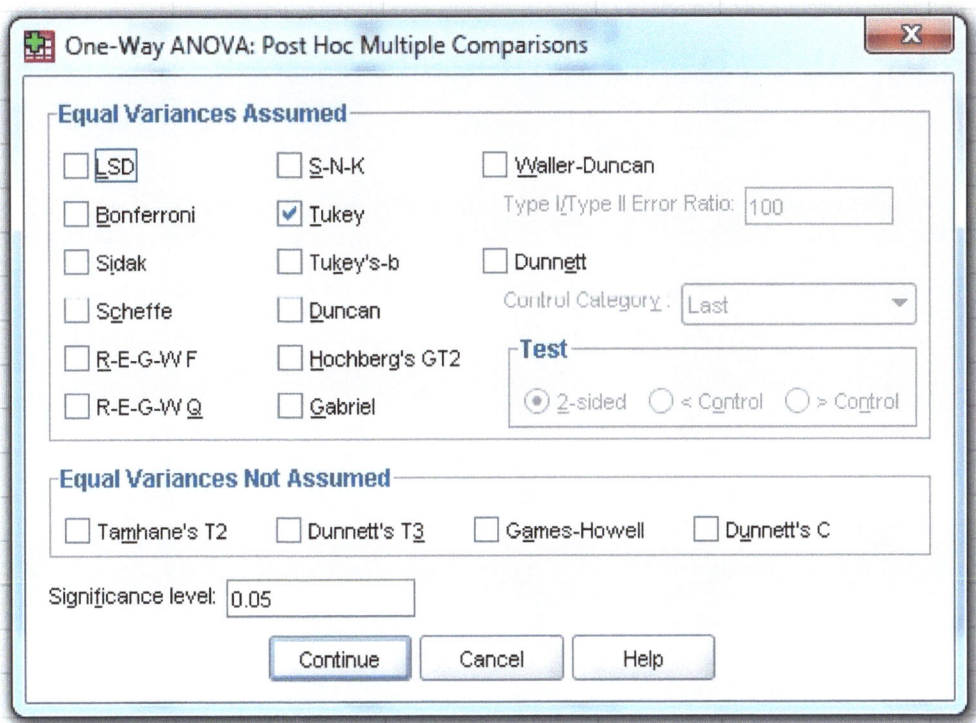

Then click continue ------------------------ Then click the Options button

Tick the Descriptive checkbox in the Statistics area. Tick Means plot

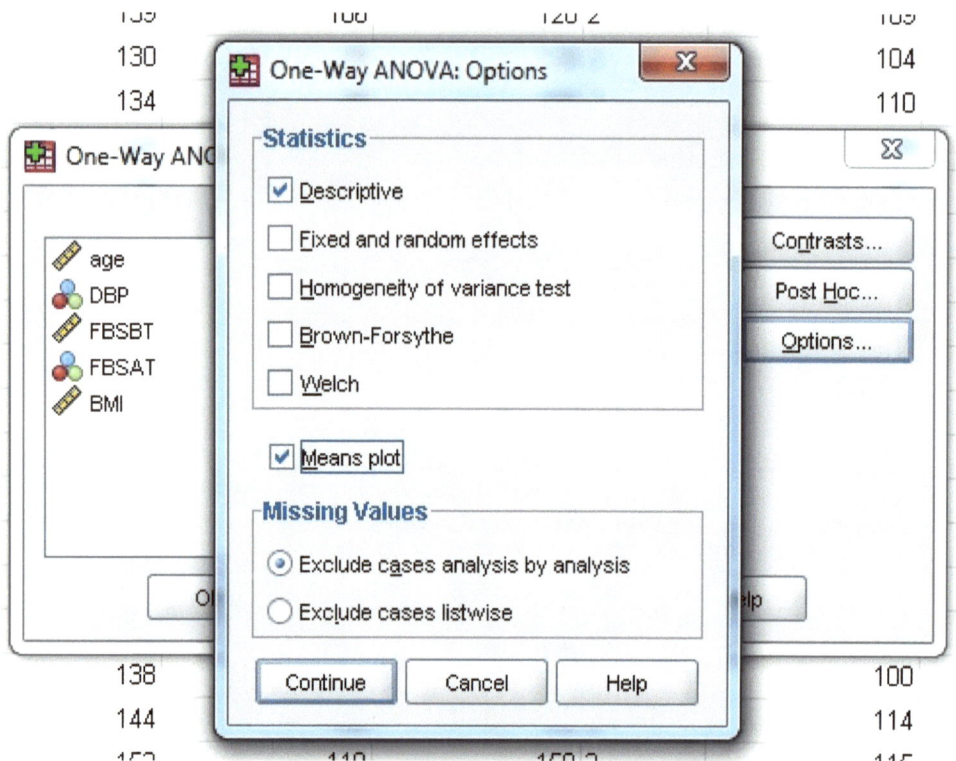

Click Continue ---------------------- Click OK

The results appears in Output window as follows.

Descriptives

SBP

	N	Mean	Std. Deviation	Std. Error	95% Confidence Interval for Mean		Minimum	Maximum
					Lower Bound	Upper Bound		
malay	17	139.12	4.675	1.134	136.71	141.52	126	145
chinese	6	133.50	9.418	3.845	123.62	143.38	122	146
indians	14	140.14	7.368	1.969	135.89	144.40	128	152
others	3	133.67	1.528	.882	129.87	137.46	132	135
Total	40	138.23	6.727	1.064	136.07	140.38	122	152

First table shows the description of continuous variable (here systolic blood pressure) in each groups of the categorical variable (here ethnicity).

Next is the ANOVA table which shows if the difference in means of continuous variable in different groups of categorical variable is statistically significant

ANOVA

SBP

	Sum of Squares	df	Mean Square	F	Sig.
Between Groups	261.329	3	87.110	2.086	.119
Within Groups	1503.646	36	41.768		
Total	1764.975	39			

If Sig. value is <0.05, the difference in means is statistically significant.

Check for Multiple comparison table

Multiple Comparisons

SBP
Tukey HSD

(I) race	(J) race	Mean Difference (I-J)	Std. Error	Sig.	95% Confidence Interval	
					Lower Bound	Upper Bound
malay	chinese	5.618	3.069	.276	-2.65	13.88
	indians	-1.025	2.332	.971	-7.31	5.26
	others	5.451	4.047	.540	-5.45	16.35
chinese	malay	-5.618	3.069	.276	-13.88	2.65
	indians	-6.643	3.154	.170	-15.14	1.85
	others	-.167	4.570	1.000	-12.47	12.14
indians	malay	1.025	2.332	.971	-5.26	7.31
	chinese	6.643	3.154	.170	-1.85	15.14
	others	6.476	4.112	.405	-4.60	17.55
others	malay	-5.451	4.047	.540	-16.35	5.45
	chinese	.167	4.570	1.000	-12.14	12.47
	indians	-6.476	4.112	.405	-17.55	4.60

The above table show the difference between means of each groups, 95% confidence interval of difference between means of each groups and Sig. value. If Sig. value is <0.05, the difference in means is statistically significant for that pair of groups.

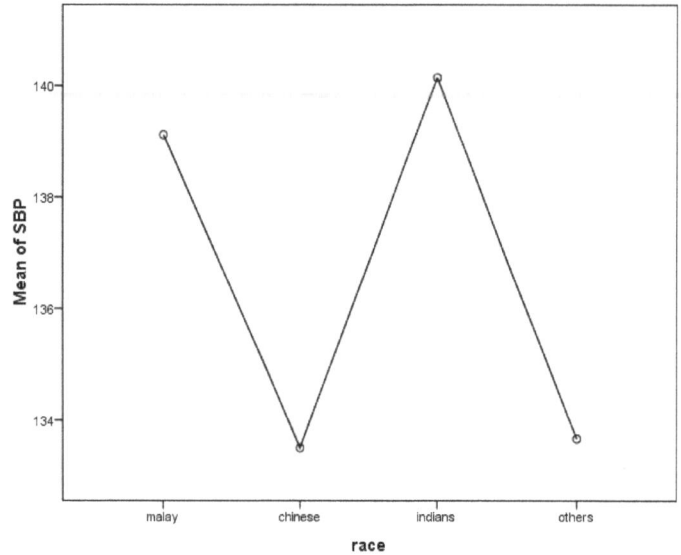

This diagram is a means plot which plots the means of different groups.

Interpretation of 1 way ANOVA in the given example

There was no statistically significant difference in systolic blood pressure between different ethnic groups as determined by one-way ANOVA ($F = 2.086$, $p = .119$). A Tukey post-hoc test revealed that there were no statistically significant differences between each ethnic groups.

Chapter 6

Non parametric tests using SPSS

The pre requisites for doing a non-parametric test are as follows.

- Comparison of means between 2 or more groups
- Continuous variable should be of interval or ratio scale
- Data is not normally distributed / skewed
- Variance in different groups are not equal

Different non parametric tests are

1. Wilcoxon Signed Rank test
2. Mann Whitney U Test
3. Kruskal Wallis Test

How to do Mann Whitney U Test

Mann Whitney U Test is applied to compare a continuous variable in two independent groups. It is an alternative to Independent Samples T test when the data is not normally distributed.

Analyze ------- Non parametric Tests ---------- 2 Independent Samples

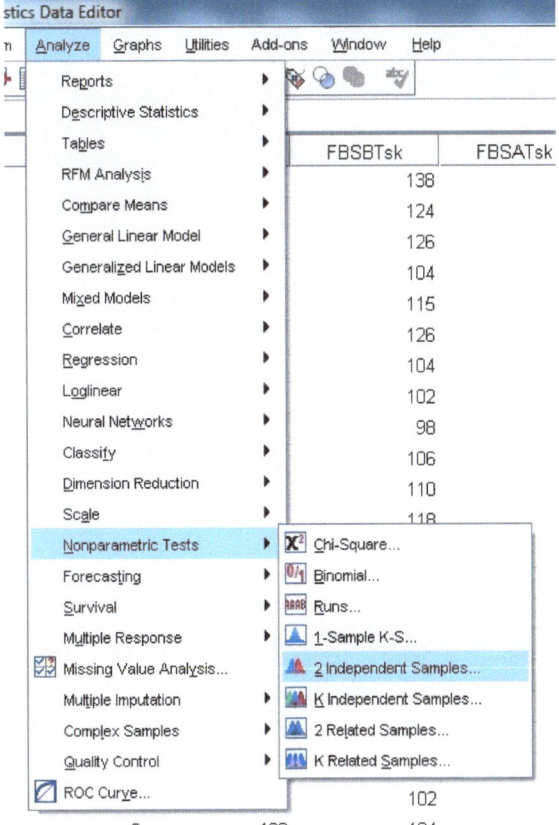

A window appears like this

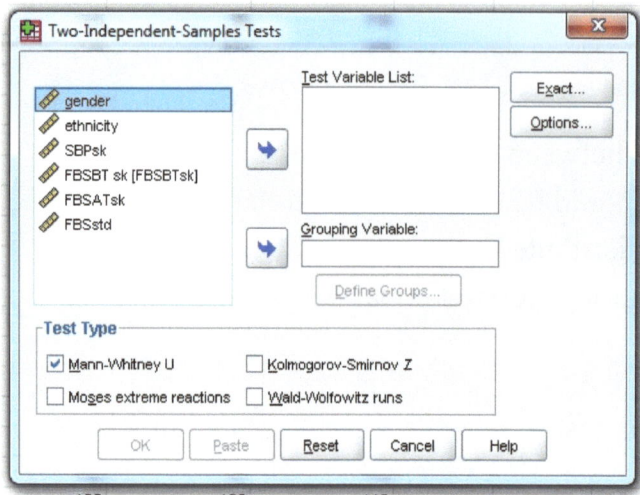

Select the continuous variable to the Test variable list and dichotomous categorical variable to the grouping variable. Make sure that grouping variable is having only 2 categories (make sure that it is a dichotomous variable). Then click check box for Mann Whitney U.

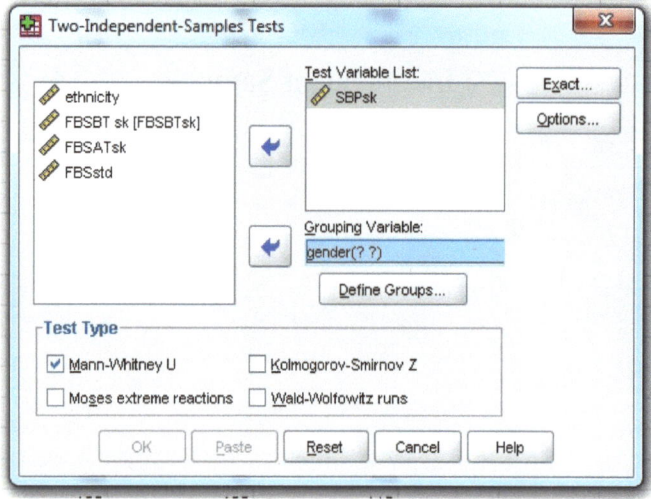

Click define groups ------------------------- Give numbers 1 and 2 for group 1 and group 2 respectively.

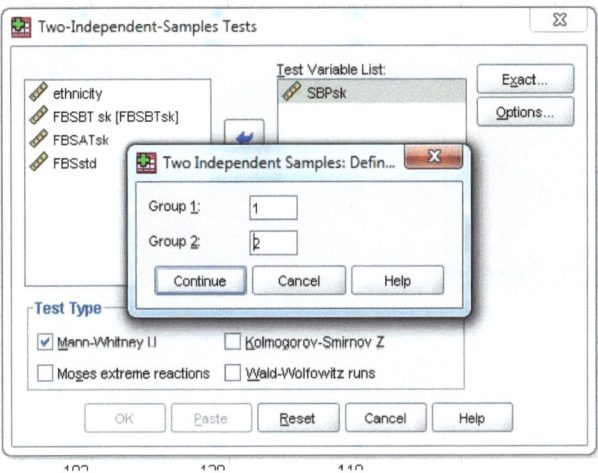

Click Continue ---------------------- Click Options

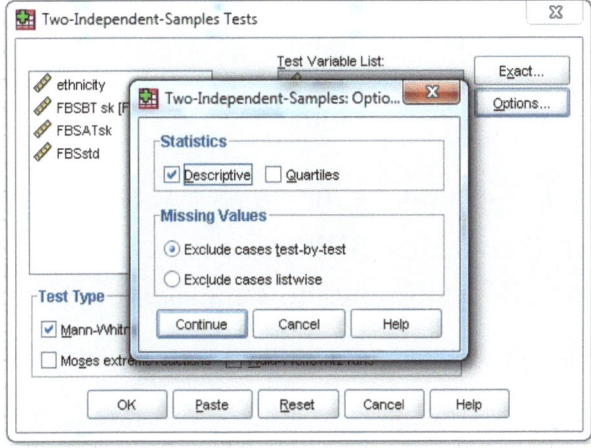

Select checkbox for Descriptive -------------------------- Click Continue -----------
------------------- Click Ok

The results appears in Output window as follows.

MANN WHITNEY U TEST

Ranks

	gender	N	Mean Rank	Sum of Ranks
SBPsk	1	18	21.08	379.50
	2	22	20.02	440.50
	Total	40		

Test Statistics[b]

	SBPsk
Mann-Whitney U	187.500
Wilcoxon W	440.500
Z	-.286
Asymp. Sig. (2-tailed)	.775
Exact Sig. [2*(1-tailed Sig.)]	.778[a]

a. Not corrected for ties.

b. Grouping Variable: gender

Interpretation of result – Z statistic in this example is -0.286 and Asymptotic Sig. value (P value) is >0.05. This means that median SBP value among males is not significantly different from median SBP value among females.

How to do Wilcoxon Signed Rank Test

Wilcoxon Signed Rank Test is applied to compare a continuous variable in two related groups. It is an alternative to Paired Samples T test when the data is not normally distributed.

Analyze ---------- Non parametric Tests ------------------ 2 Related Samples

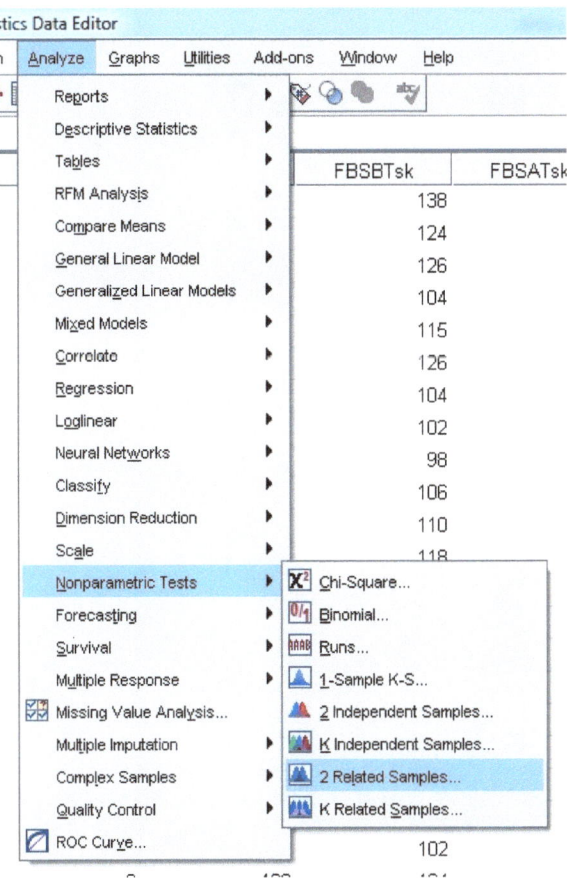

A window appears like this

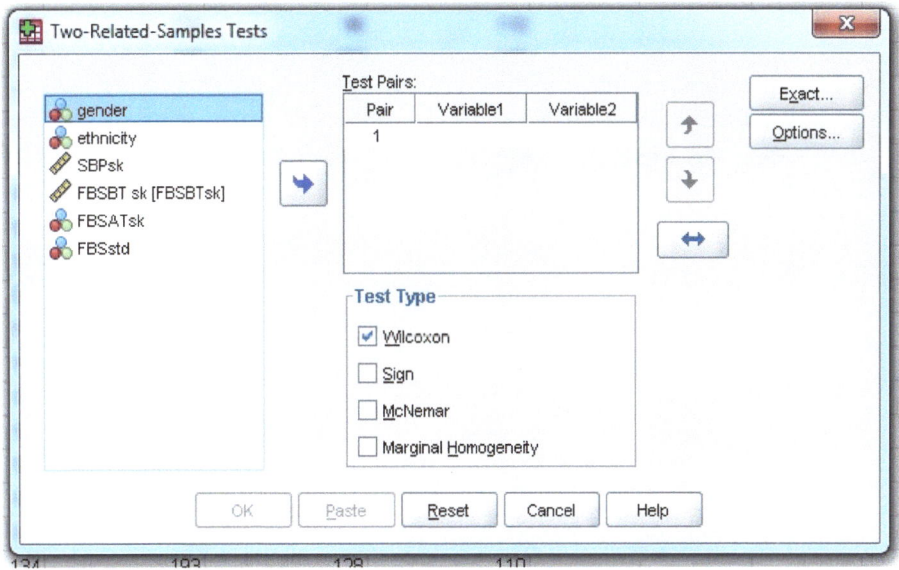

Select the paired continuous variable (eg:- FBS before treatment and FBS after treatment) to the Test Pairs and tick checkbox for Wilcoxon.

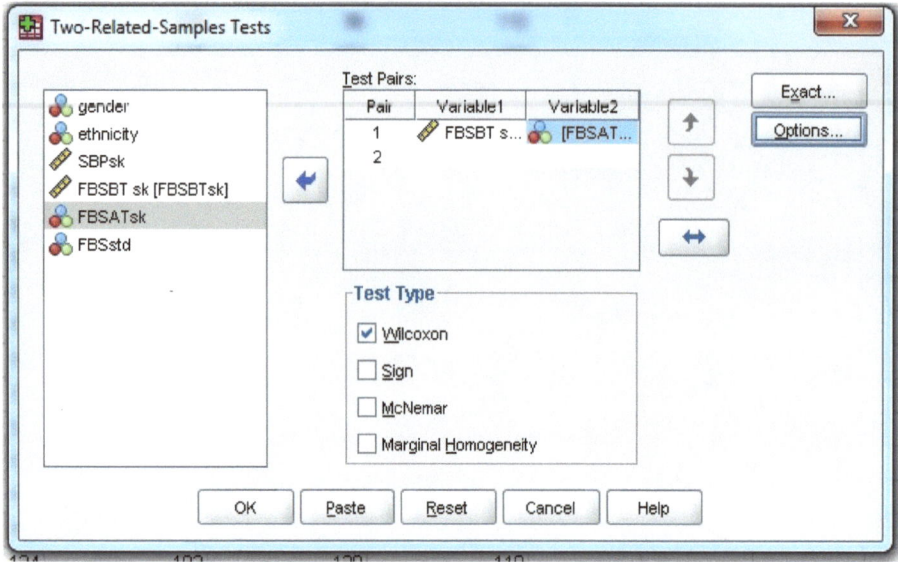

Click Options and click Descriptive

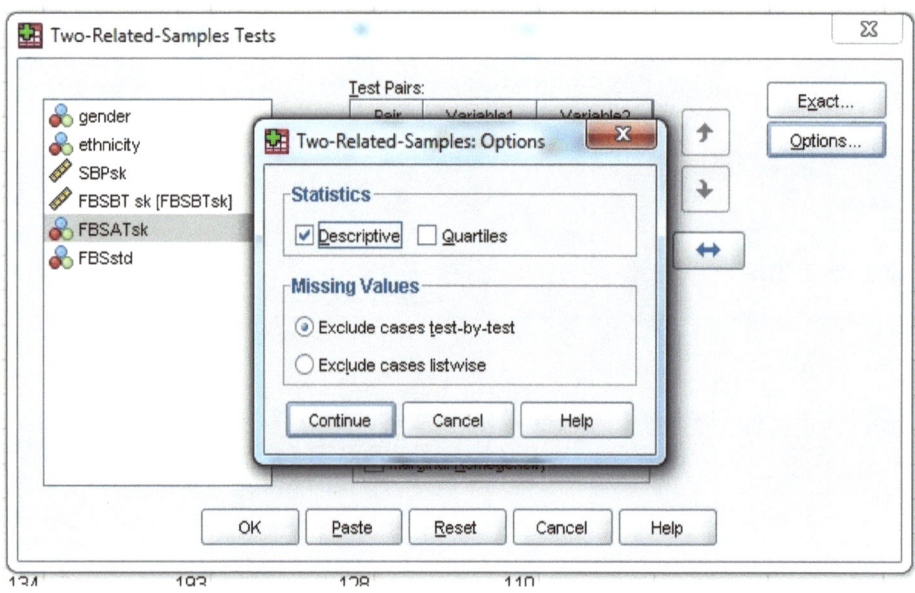

Select checkbox for Descriptive ------- Click Continue ------ Click OK

The results appears in Output window as follows.

Descriptive Statistics

	N	Mean	Std. Deviation	Minimum	Maximum
FBSBT sk	40	125.45	28.597	92	228
FBSATsk	40	106.45	11.710	91	138

Wilcoxon Signed Ranks Test

Ranks

		N	Mean Rank	Sum of Ranks
FBSATsk - FBSBT sk	Negative Ranks	35[a]	21.93	767.50
	Positive Ranks	5[b]	10.50	52.50
	Ties	0[c]		
	Total	40		

a. FBSATsk < FBSBT sk

b. FBSATsk > FBSBT sk

c. FBSATsk = FBSBT sk

Test Statistics[b]

	FBSATsk - FBSBT sk
Z	-4.806[a]
Asymp. Sig. (2-tailed)	.000

a. Based on positive ranks.

b. Wilcoxon Signed Ranks Test

Interpretation of result – Z statistic in this example is -4.806 and Asymptotic Sig. value (P value) is <0.05. This means that median FBS value before treatment is significantly different from median FBS value after treatment.

Kruskal Wallis Test – is applied to test if the difference in mean values of a continuous variable between more than 2 different groups is statistically significant. This test is a non-parametric test, which is applied when the data is not normally distributed.

One variable is a continuous variable and the other variable is a categorical variable having more than 2 categories.

How to do Kruskal Wallis test

Analyze ---------- Non Parametric--------------------K Independent Samples

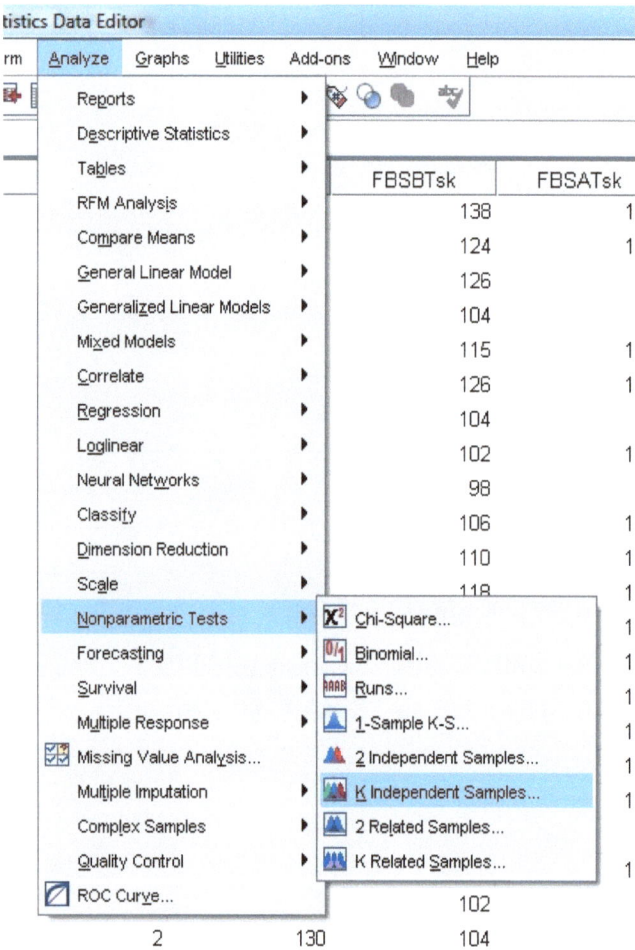

Then the following window appears

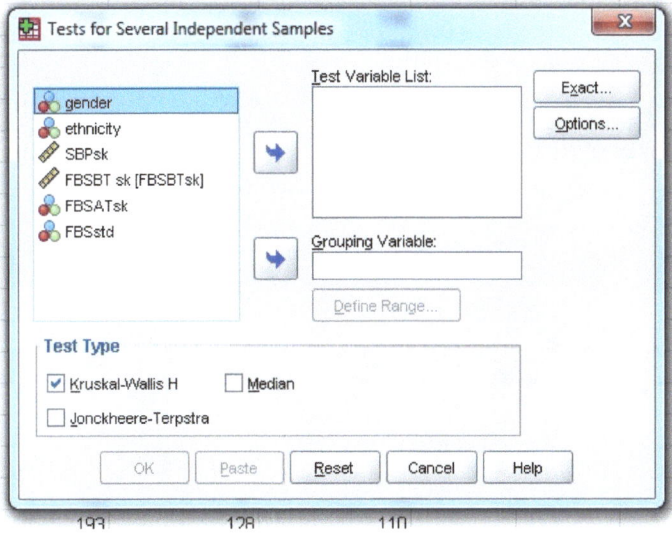

Select the continuous variable in Test Variable List and the categorical variable as Grouping Variable.

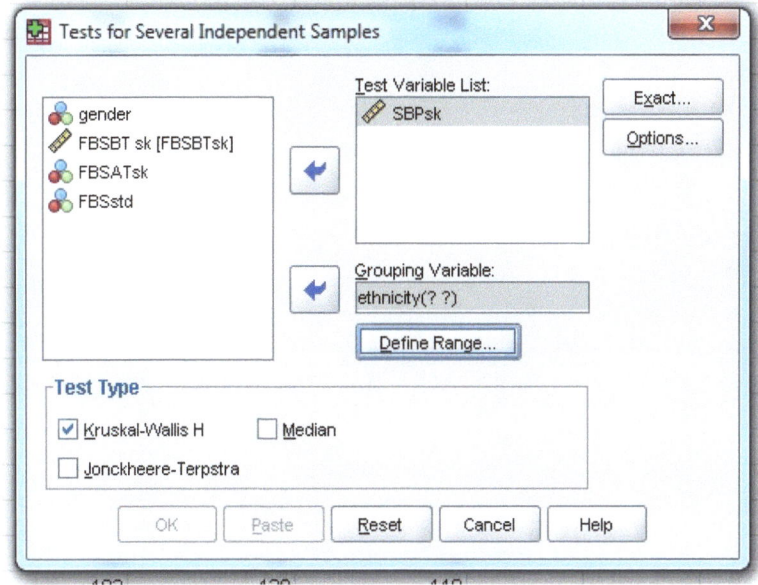

Click Define Range and give the range of grouping of the categorical variable. In this example there are 4 groups for ethnicity (1 – malay, 2 – Chinese, 3 – Indian and 4 – others).

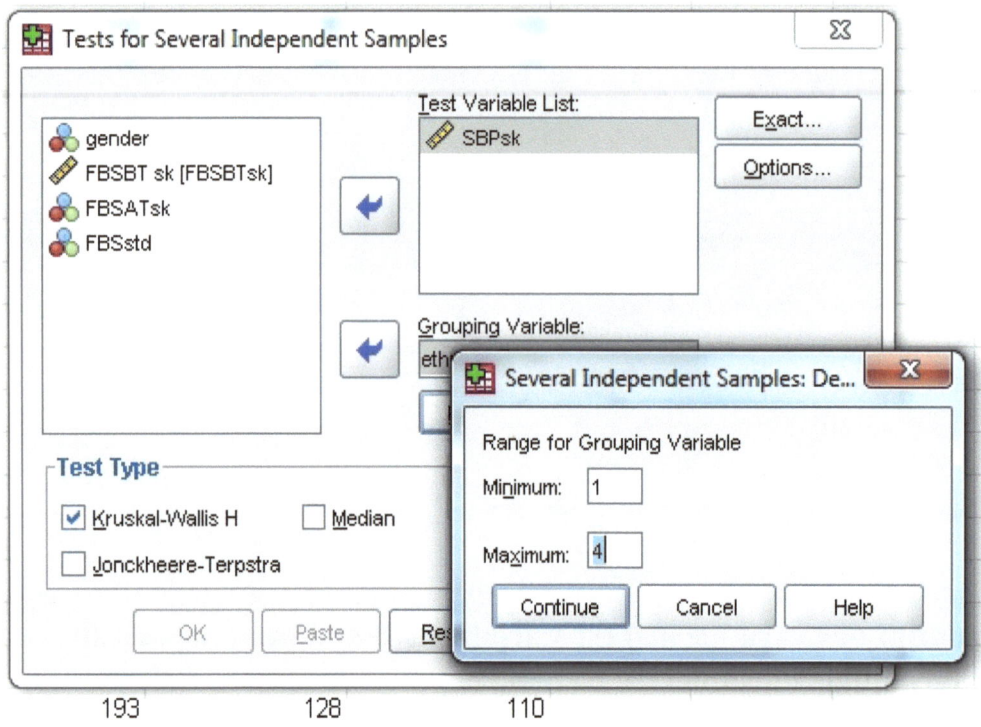

Give Range for Grouping Variable ---------------------------- Click Continue

Then Click Options

Then Tick checkbox for Descriptive ---------------------------Then Click Continue

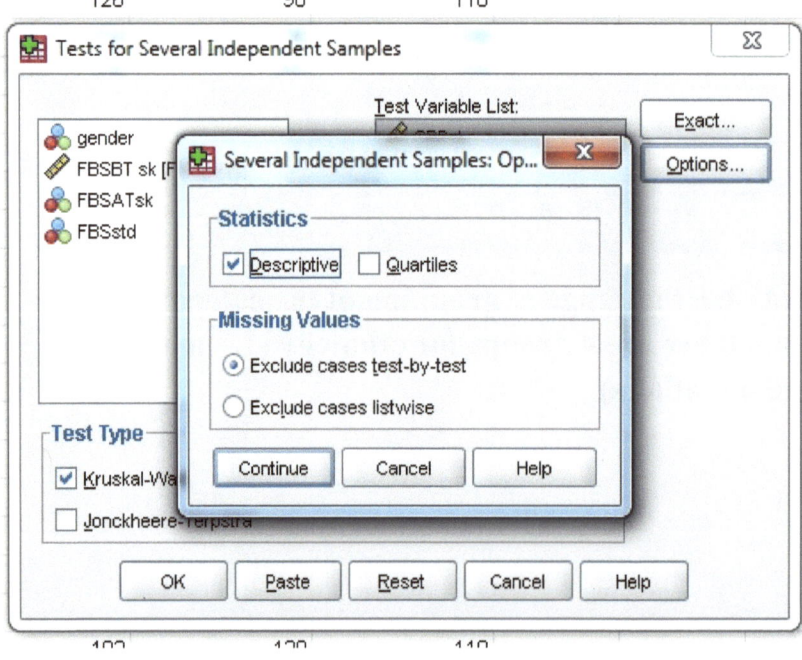

Then Tick checkbox for Kruskal Wallis H

Then click OK

The results appears in Output window as follows.

Kruskal-Wallis Test

Ranks

	ethnicity	N	Mean Rank
SBPsk	1	17	20.62
	2	6	24.75
	3	14	19.79
	4	3	14.67
	Total	40	

Test Statistics[a,b]

	SBPsk
Chi-Square	1.599
df	3
Asymp. Sig.	.660

a. Kruskal Wallis Test

b. Grouping Variable: ethnicity

Interpretation of Kruskal Wallis Test in the given example

There was no statistically significant difference in systolic blood pressure between different ethnic groups as determined by Kruskal Wallis Test (*Asymptotic Sig. value* = .660).

Chapter 7

Correlation Analysis using SPSS

Correlation shows the linear relationship between 2 continuous variables.

2 types of Correlation analysis are

a.   Pearson's Correlation – used when both of the continuous variables are normally distributed

b.   Spearman's correlation – used when either one or both of the continuous variables are not normally distributed

How to do Correlation Analysis

Analyse ---------------- Correlate ----------------------- Bivariate

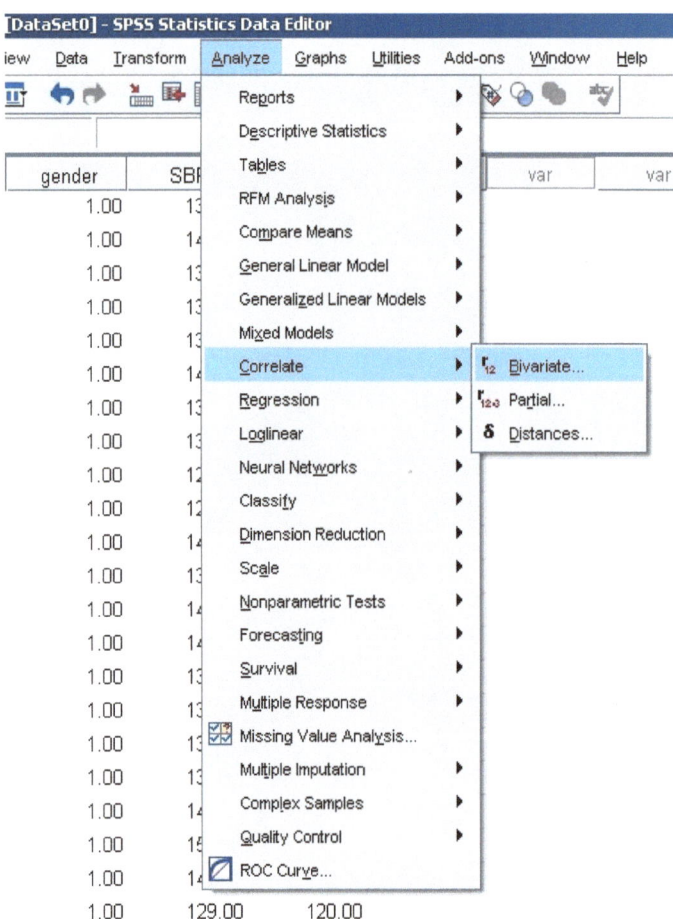

Then select the continuous variables, whose correlation is to be analyzed

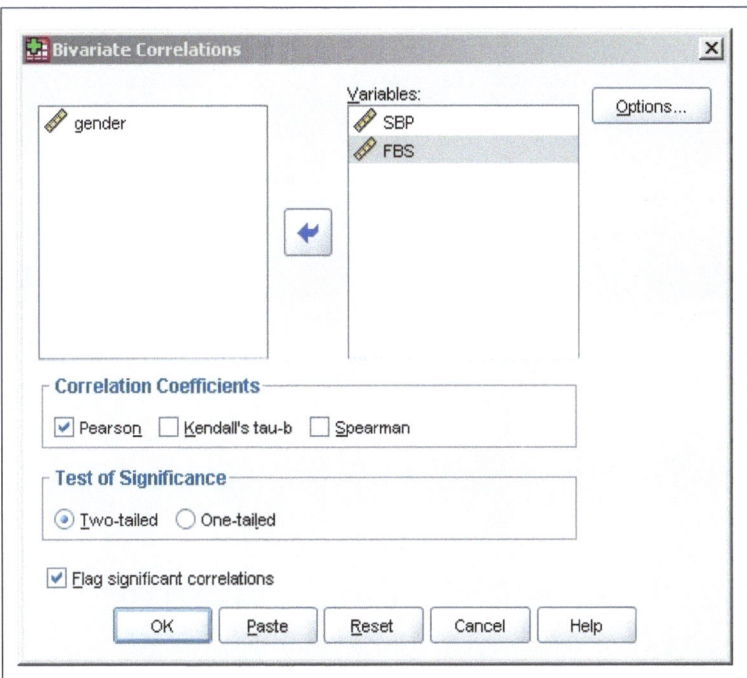

Select Pearson Correlation coefficient (when data is normally distributed), or Spearman's Correlation coefficient (when data is not normally distributed.

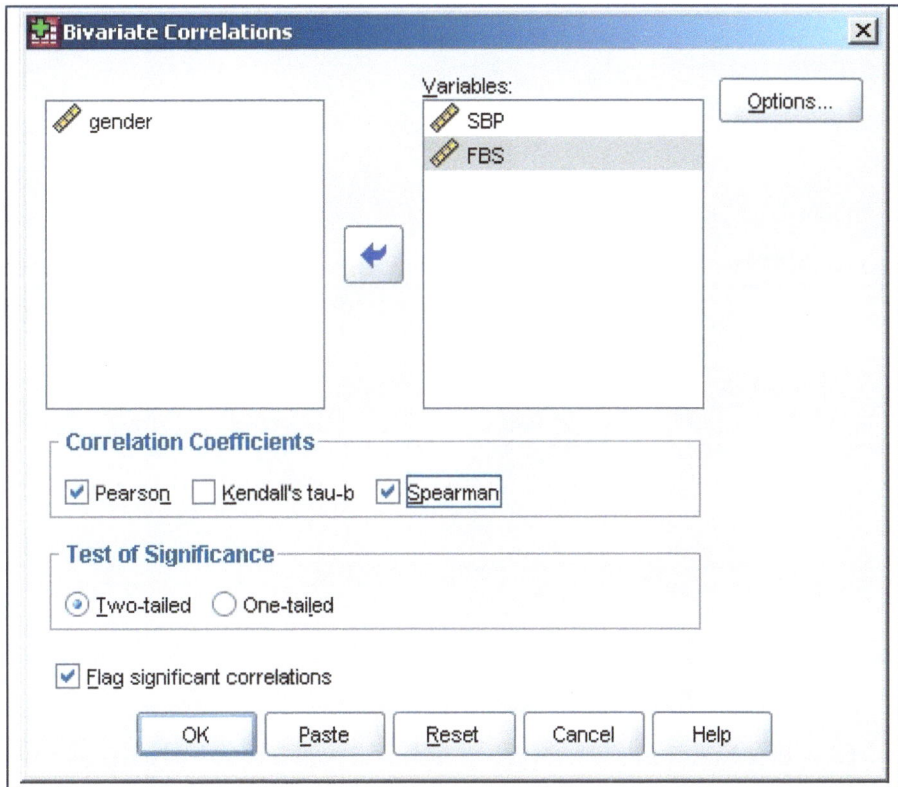

Click OK

The results appear in output window as follows

Correlations

Correlations

		SBP	FBS
SBP	Pearson Correlation	1	.510**
	Sig. (2-tailed)		.001
	N	40	40
FBS	Pearson Correlation	.510**	1
	Sig. (2-tailed)	.001	
	N	40	40

**. Correlation is significant at the 0.01 level (2-tailed).

This analysis shows that the Pearson correlation coefficient is 0.510. That means that there is a positive correlation between Systolic Blood Pressure and Fasting Blood Sugar. The Sig. value or P value is 0.001. That means that correlation is statistically significant.

Nonparametric Correlations

Correlations

			SBP	FBS
Spearman's rho	SBP	Correlation Coefficient	1.000	.575**
		Sig. (2-tailed)	.	.000
		N	40	40
	FBS	Correlation Coefficient	.575**	1.000
		Sig. (2-tailed)	.000	.
		N	40	40

**. Correlation is significant at the 0.01 level (2-tailed).

The result of non parametric correlation or Spearman's correlation shows that the Spearman's rank correlation coefficient (pronounced in greek as Spearman's rho) is 0.575. That means that there is a positive correlation between Systolic Blood Pressure and Fasting Blood Sugar. The Sig. value or P value is 0.000. That means that correlation is statistically significant.

How to draw Scatter diagram with line of fit for correlation analysis

In the previous example for correlation between Systolic Blood Pressure and Fasting Blood Sugar, we can draw a scatter diagram using SPSS.

Click Graphs ----------- Chart Builder

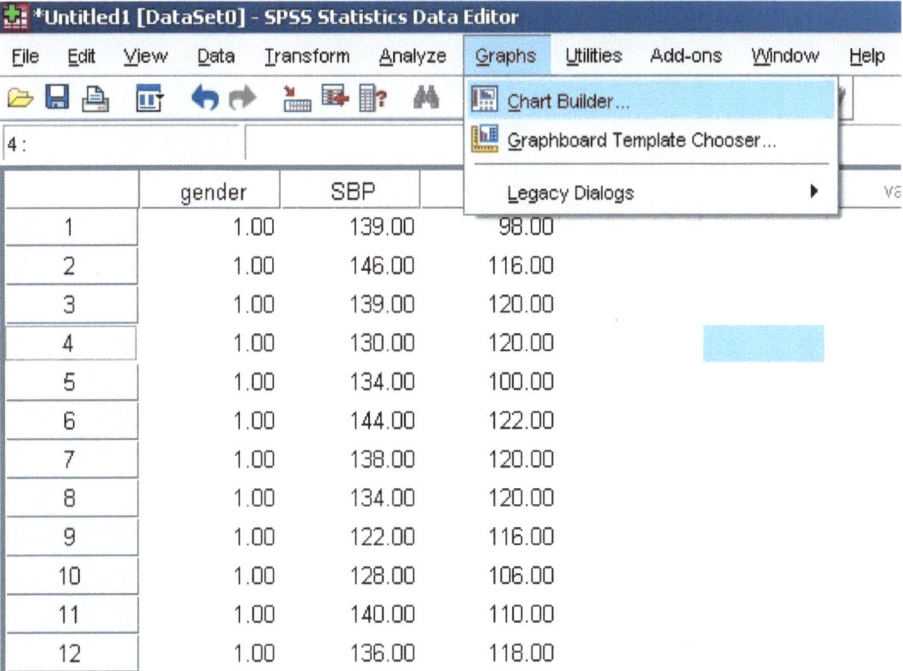

Then following message box appears.

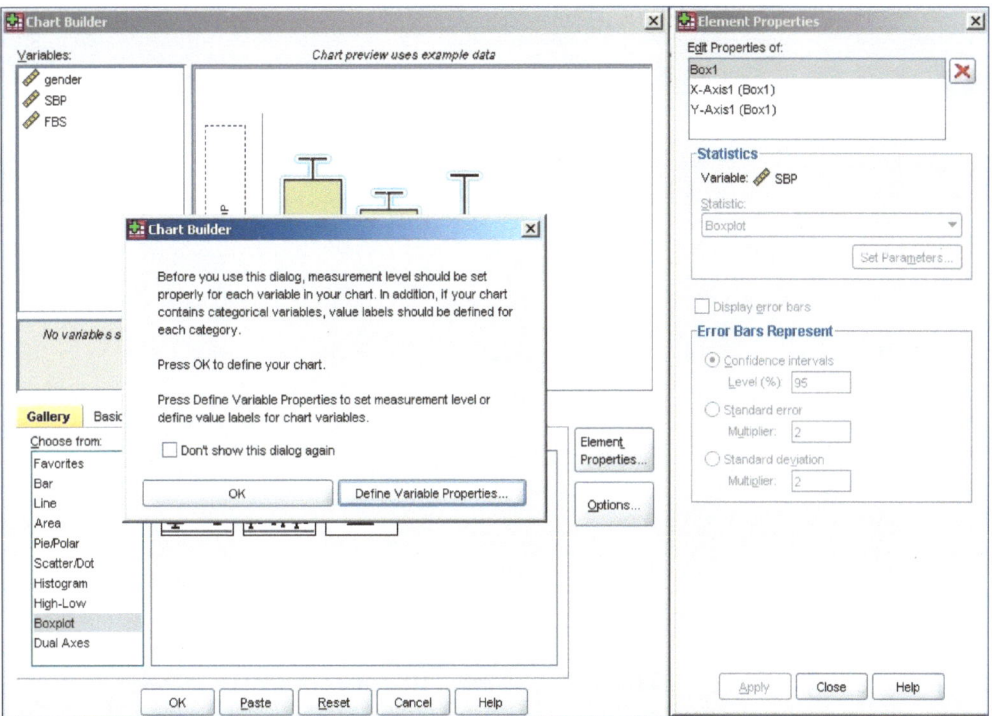

Click OK

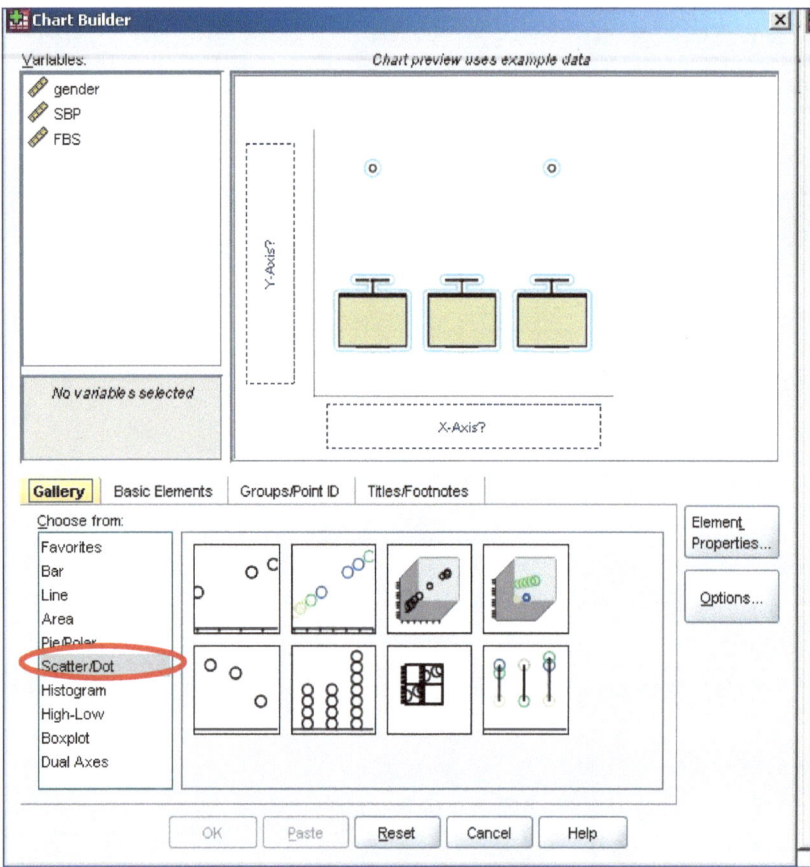

Click Gallery

Then Choose from Scatter / Dot

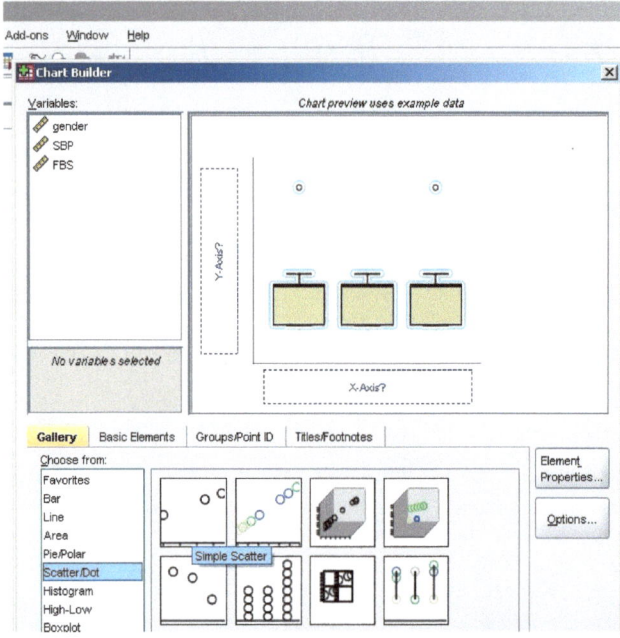

Then select Simple Scatter and drag to the chart preview area. Then it appears like below.

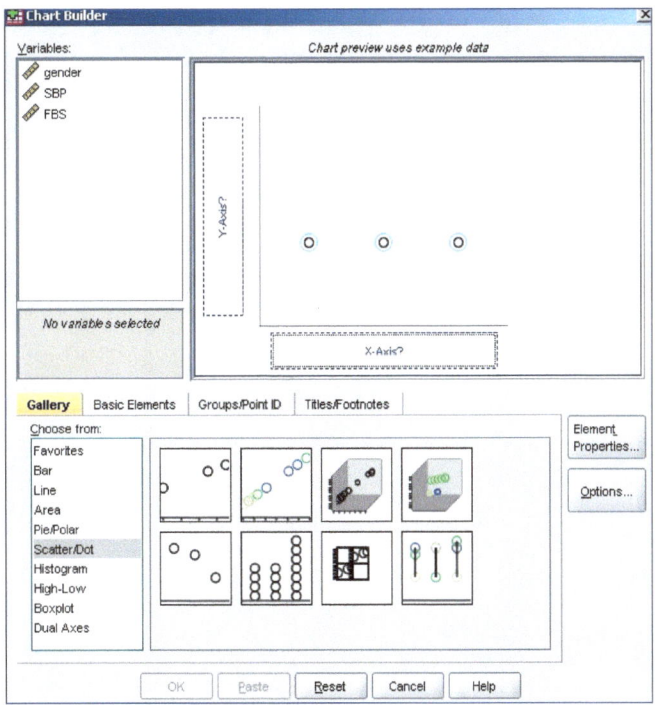

Then you drag the variables to X axis and Y axis as required.

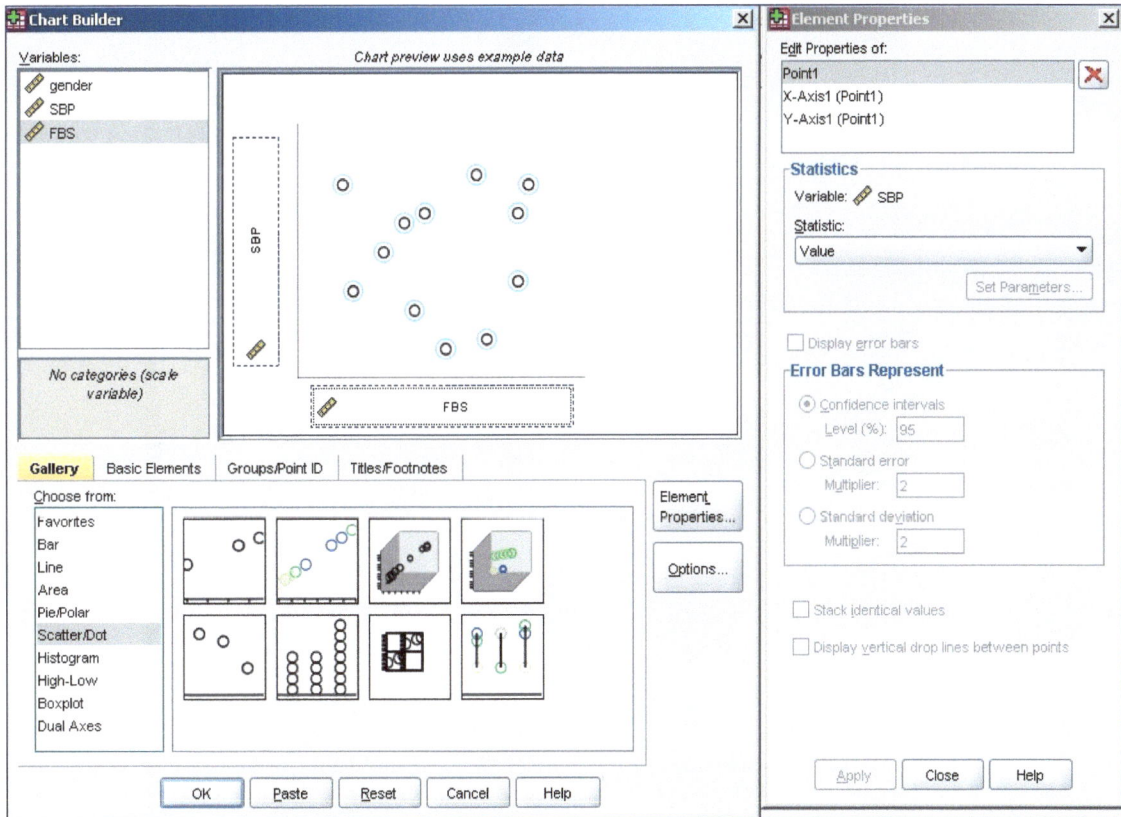

Here I dragged FBS to X axis and SBP to Y axis.

Now you have to edit Element properties on the box on the right side.

Select Y axis1 on the element properties,

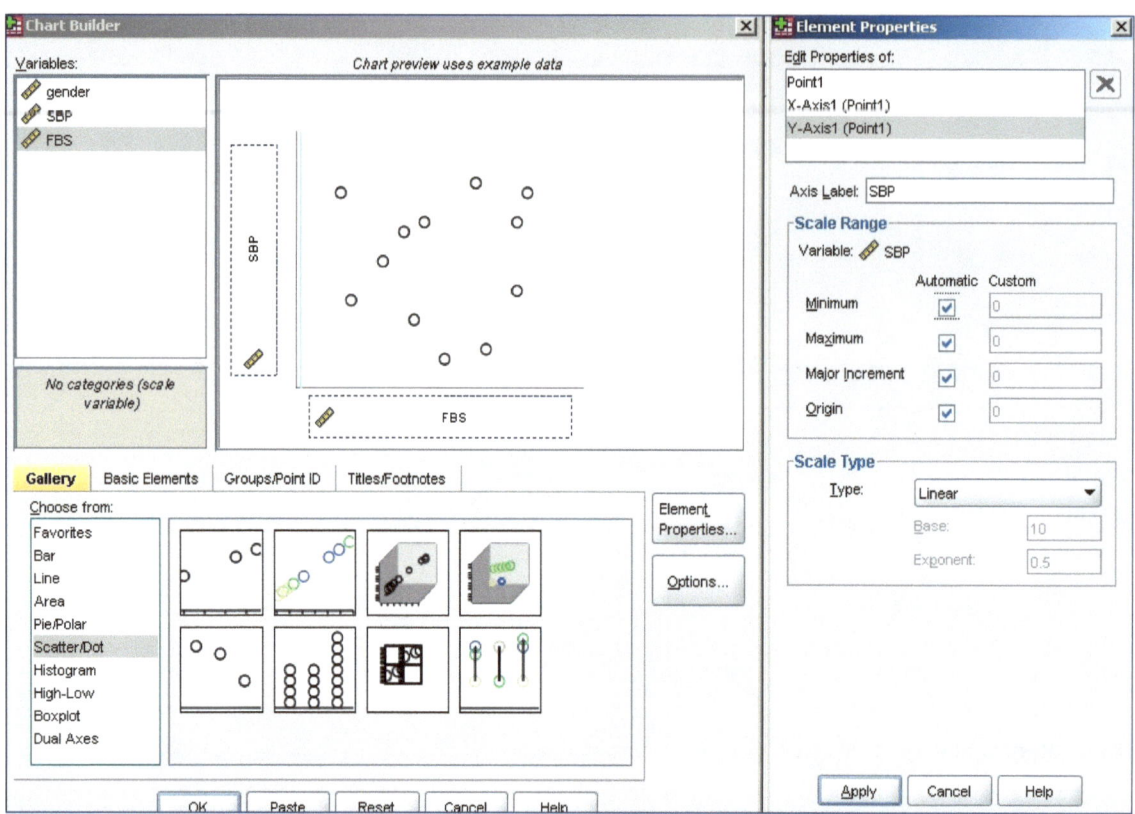

Then change Minimum of Y axis1 from automatic to Custom and keep the value as 0.

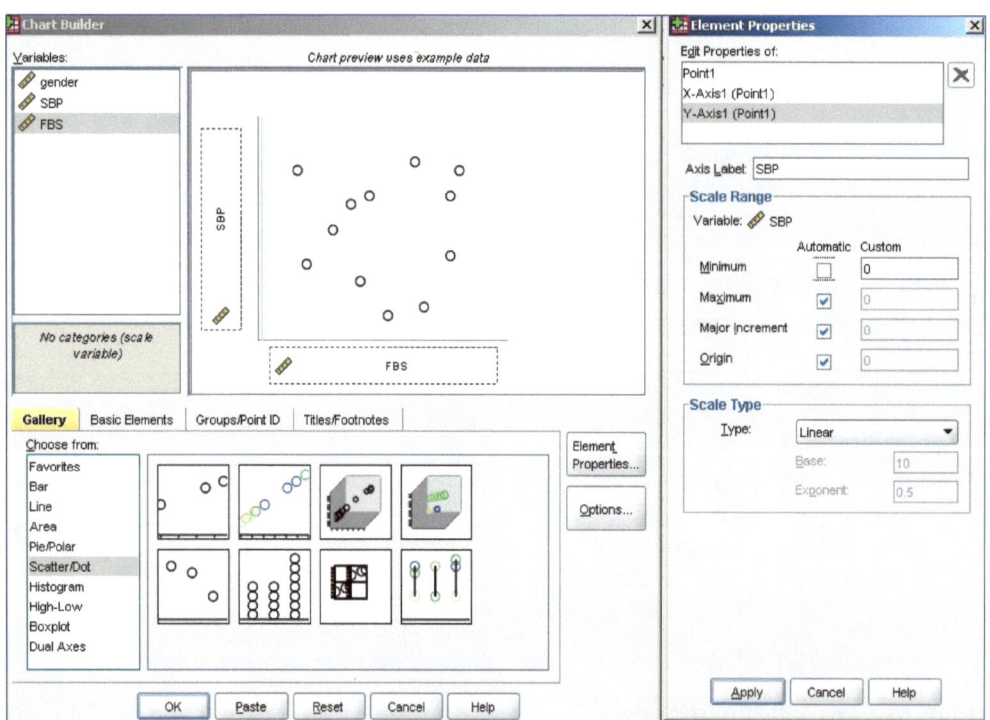

Then apply and Click OK

Then scatter / dot plot appears in output view as follows

GGraph

[DataSet0]

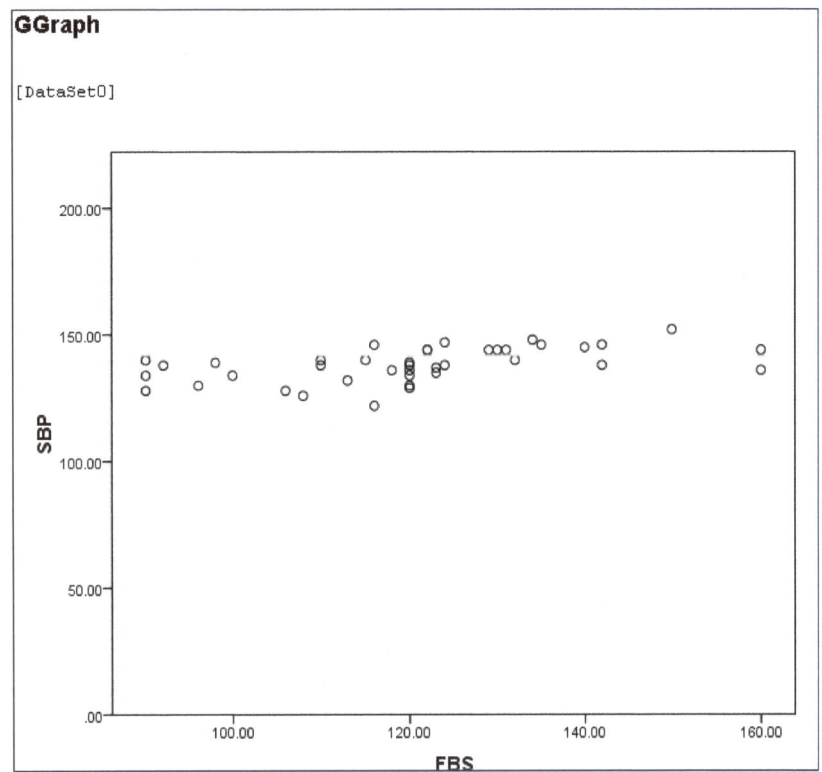

To put line of fit, you have to double click the diagram

Then diagram opens in chart editor view

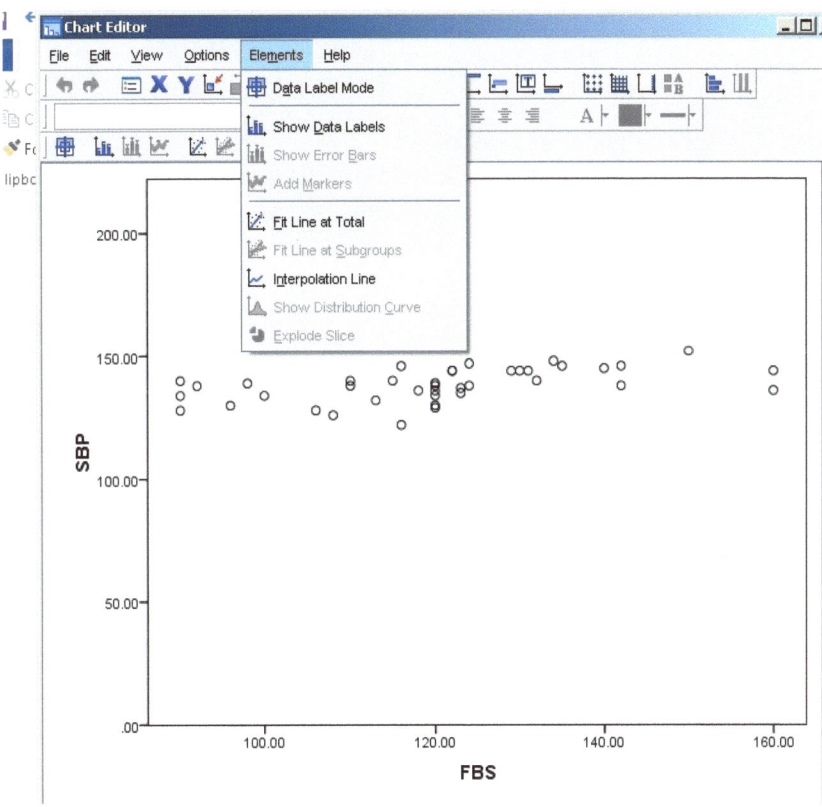

Click on Elements in menu and click Fit line at total. Then fitline appears.

You can select linear fit line

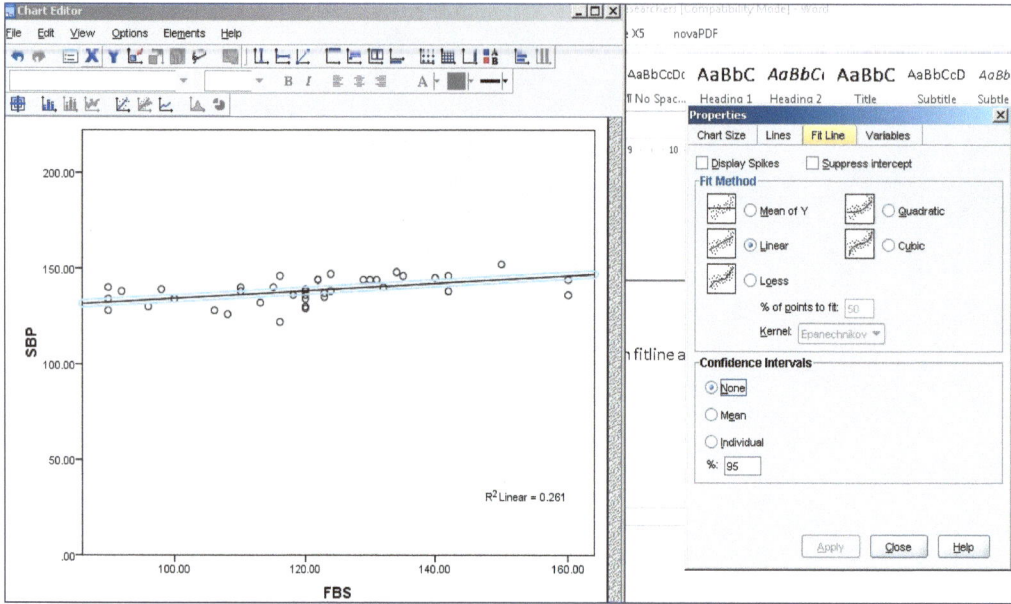

R^2 value appears. In this example R^2 value is 0.261. It is the coefficient of determination. That means that 26.1% of the dependent variable (here SBP) can be predicted from the independent variable (here FBS).

www.ingramcontent.com/pod-product-compliance
Lightning Source LLC
Chambersburg PA
CBHW050733180526

45159CB00003B/1212